Patient Care Guidelines for Family Nurse Practitioners

Patient Care Guidelines for Family Nurse Practitioners

Edited by

Axalla J. Hoole, M.D.

Assistant Professor of Medicine,
The University of North Carolina School of Medicine;
Assistant Attending Physician,
Department of Medicine,
North Carolina Memorial Hospital,
Chapel Hill, North Carolina

Robert A. Greenberg, M.D.

Assistant Professor of Pediatrics,
The University of North Carolina School of Medicine;
Assistant Attending Physician,
Department of Pediatrics,
North Carolina Memorial Hospital,
Chapel Hill, North Carolina

C. Glenn Pickard, Jr., M.D.

Associate Professor of Medicine,
The University of North Carolina School of Medicine;
Associate Attending Physician,
Department of Medicine,
North Carolina Memorial Hospital,
Chapel Hill, North Carolina

Little, Brown and Company   Boston

Library of Congress Catalog Card No. 75-30284

ISBN 0-316-372218

Printed in the United States of America

Contributing Authors

James R. Dingfelder, M.D.
Assistant Professor of Obstetrics and Gynecology,
The University of North Carolina School of Medicine;
Assistant Attending Physician,
Department of Obstetrics and Gynecology,
North Carolina Memorial Hospital,
Chapel Hill, North Carolina

Robert A. Greenberg, M.D.
Assistant Professor of Pediatrics,
The University of North Carolina School of Medicine;
Assistant Attending Physician,
Department of Pediatrics,
North Carolina Memorial Hospital,
Chapel Hill, North Carolina

Harvey J. Hamrick, M.D.
Assistant Professor of Pediatrics,
The University of North Carolina School of Medicine;
Assistant Attending Physician,
Department of Pediatrics,
North Carolina Memorial Hospital,
Chapel Hill, North Carolina

Axalla J. Hoole, M.D.
Assistant Professor of Medicine,
The University of North Carolina School of Medicine;
Assistant Attending Physician,
Department of Medicine,
North Carolina Memorial Hospital,
Chapel Hill, North Carolina

Robert S. Lawrence, M.D.
Assistant Professor of Medicine and
Director of the Harvard Primary Care Program,
Harvard Medical School;
Acting Chief of Medicine,
Cambridge Hospital,
Cambridge, Massachusetts

Gregory S. Liptak, M.D., M.P.H.
Pediatrician,
National Health Service Corps,
Aurora, New York

Frank A. Loda, M.D.
Associate Professor of Pediatrics,
The University of North Carolina School of Medicine;
Associate Attending Physician,
Department of Pediatrics,
North Carolina Memorial Hospital,
Chapel Hill, North Carolina

Jack P. Mercer, M.D.
Associate Professor of Obstetrics and Gynecology,
The University of North Carolina School of Medicine;
Associate Attending Physician,
Department of Obstetrics and Gynecology,
North Carolina Memorial Hospital,
Chapel Hill, North Carolina

C. Glenn Pickard, Jr., M.D.
Associate Professor of Medicine,
The University of North Carolina School of Medicine;
Associate Attending Physician,
Department of Medicine,
North Carolina Memorial Hospital,
Chapel Hill, North Carolina

Samuel M. Putnam, M.D.
Assistant Professor of Medicine,
The University of North Carolina School of Medicine;
Assistant Attending Physician,
Department of Medicine,
North Carolina Memorial Hospital,
Chapel Hill, North Carolina

Contributing Authors

Contributing Authors

James E. Schwankl, M.D., M.P.H.
Instructor of Pediatrics,
    The University of North Carolina School of Medicine;
        Assistant Attending Physician,
            Department of Pediatrics,
                North Carolina Memorial Hospital,
                    Chapel Hill, North Carolina

Fred D. Summers, M.D.
Assistant Professor of Obstetrics and Gynecology,
    The University of North Carolina School of Medicine;
        Assistant Attending Physician,
            Department of Obstetrics and Gynecology,
                North Carolina Memorial Hospital,
                    Chapel Hill, North Carolina

Edward H. Wagner, M.D., M.P.H.
Assistant Professor of Medicine and Epidemiology,
    The University of North Carolina School of Medicine
    and School of Public Health;
        Assistant Attending Physician,
            Department of Medicine,
                North Carolina Memorial Hospital,
                    Chapel Hill, North Carolina

Nelson A. Warner, M.D.
Dermatologist,
    Private Practice,
        Winter Haven, Florida

Preface

In the decade from 1965 to the present, the United States has been faced with a major problem in the quantity, quality, and accessibility of health care services. This problem has affected primary health care services generally and has been particularly acute both in the inner city and in rural areas. The disappearance of the "crossroads" general practitioner from the small towns and villages of the rural areas and the flight of physicians from the inner cities to the suburbs have created problems in health care delivery, which have stimulated a wide variety of programs designed to meet the resultant health care crisis.

As one response to this crisis, the Schools of Nursing, Public Health, and Medicine of the University of North Carolina at Chapel Hill have collaboratively developed a training program for family nurse practitioners (FNPs). Now in its sixth year, the program has trained 110 FNPs for practice in North Carolina. In conjunction with the training program, faculty members of the schools have participated in innovative primary health care delivery programs in which FNPs staff satellite clinics, with physicians serving as consultants and supervisors for their medical practice.

The patient care guidelines developed for the training program and used in the demonstration practice are presented in this book. They have been revised many times and are still being revised to reflect new practices and the changing role of nurse practitioners. They remain relatively arbitrary and dogmatic. They are not intended as an exhaustive treatise on the illnesses covered nor as an exposition of all the ways each illness may be managed. Rather, they are intended to codify an acceptable set of criteria for diagnosing a particular condition and to present an acceptable plan of management.

Despite their limitations, these guidelines have proved very useful in our own practice and in the practice of other physicians and nurse practitioners in the state. We hope that by publishing them, and thus making them available to a wider audience, we may be of some assistance to others struggling with the same problems.

A. J. H.
R. A. G.
C. G. P., Jr.

Chapel Hill

Acknowledgments

We would like to acknowledge the first class of family nurse practitioners of the University of North Carolina at Chapel Hill: Evelyn Aabel, June Baise, Betty Compton, Ruth Efird, Sandra Hogan, Phoebe Hood, and Margaret Wilkman. As part of their course, they developed a set of pediatric patient care guidelines that served as a foundation for part of this book. We thank Drs. Robert Thompson and Sidney Chipman, who contributed to the early guidelines, and also our nurse practitioner and physician colleagues, who have critically reviewed many of the guidelines and offered invaluable suggestions. Finally, we extend our sincere thanks to Charlotte Spade, who has borne the major burden of the secretarial responsibility for the preparation of the manuscript.

i

Contents

Introduction: Use of Patient Care Guidelines

Several fundamental concepts underlie these patient care guidelines and need to be made clear at the outset:

1. A nurse practitioner cannot and should not engage in procedures of *medical* practice without having a defined relationship to a responsible physician who supervises the nurse's medical practice and is always available for consultation or referral from the nurse. Normal procedures of *nursing* practice, carried out by the nurse practitioner, are not under the supervision of the physician.
2. The guidelines must be thoroughly reviewed, changed if necessary, and mutually agreed to by the nurse practitioner and physician before they are implemented.
3. The patient care guidelines define the boundaries of the medical procedures available to the nurse practitioner. If there is no guideline defining a condition and its management, the nurse practitioner must not diagnose or treat the condition without direct physician involvement.
4. The nurse practitioner and responsible physician must assure one another through supervised practice that the nurse practitioner has the knowledge and skills to make the diagnosis contained in the guidelines and to render treatment as outlined. The guidelines are *not* intended to serve as a "cookbook" reference to assist in making diagnoses. Rather, they are an attempt to codify the knowledge and practices of the nurse and physician.

In settings in which we have had experience, the guidelines cover about 75 percent of the presenting problems of all patients seeking primary health care. Obviously in certain settings other conditions may occur more frequently, and the need to develop additional guidelines arises. Thus, there is a constant need to review one's practice and develop or revise guidelines.

In practice, the guidelines have been used to enable the nurse practitioner legally and ethically to engage in medical practice acts without the physician's personally seeing each patient. In certain settings the nurse and physician may be geographically separated, as when the nurse practitioner operates a satellite clinic. In this context, the guidelines are often referred to as *standing orders*. When they are used in this manner, the nurse practitioner indicates for each condition treated the appropriate guideline followed. The clinical note should contain adequate information to assure anyone reading it that the patient's condition fits the guideline being followed. In practice, the nurse practitioner needs to refer to the guidelines for common conditions only as a check; the condition being managed and the correct procedures usually are known before checking with the guidelines.

An additional use of the guidelines is as a standard of care in medical audit procedures. To be used effectively in this manner, however, demands that the practitioners being audited have an opportunity to review, discuss, and modify the guidelines *before* any audit begins in order to ensure that they are appropriate standards for the geographic area and the specific practi

We are not presumptuous enough to assert that the guidelines that we hav developed are of immediate or widespread applicability as standards of care. They should simply serve as a point of departure from which to develop guid lines that suit local norms and conditions.

A final word regarding the format is in order. Originally we experimented with clinical algorhythms or branching logic trees. While we found these use in attempting to analyze the clinician's approach to clinical problem-solving, found them unworkable as guides to practice. Experienced, well-trained pra titioners simply do not follow the same branching logic in dealing with each patient. The same key observations are made, but not necessarily in the sam order. We therefore abandoned that format.

We again wish to emphasize that this is, and always should remain, an un-finished work. In this regard, we welcome the comments and suggestions of others. We sincerely hope that this book will contribute to the continuing effort to provide improved patient care.

Notice

1

USE OF THE HEALTH MAINTENANCE FLOW SHEET

(Age 2 Weeks to 17 Years)

I. **Purpose of the health maintenance flow sheet (Fig. 1-1)**

   A. To guide the health care provider in recommended health maintenance procedures.

   B. To serve as a data sheet for the results of procedures.

   C. To allow the provider to individualize a patient's health maintenance program appropriately.

   D. To establish easily the relative completeness of the patient's health maintenance status.

II. **General instructions**

   A. At the patient's first health maintenance visit after registration, the recommended procedures that are appropriate for the patient's age are done (see Age-Specific Health Maintenance Guidelines [Pediatric]).

   B. The date (month and year) are recorded beside each test in the first blank column.

   C. The date of the next scheduled assessment is written in the top box of the next column (opposite the heading "Date Scheduled").

   D. Moving down the column, the boxes of the procedures to be done at the next assessment should be *outlined* by the provider with a red pencil. No other columns are marked in advance, since the purpose of outlining the procedure boxes in each column is to indicate what should be done at or before the next assessment. This can be determined only by what was actually done by the end of the previous assessment.

   E. If procedures are done before the next scheduled assessment, the date when they are done and the results are recorded in the red-outlined box.

   F. This sequence is repeated at each assessment. If a patient needs more frequent visits for health maintenance because a problem is

Procedures and Ages

Assessments 2 wk; 2, 4, 6, 9, 12, 18 mo; 2, 3, 5, 8, 11, 13, 15, 17 yr	Date scheduled														
	Date seen														
	Age														
	Provider														
Complete history	Date														
Complete examination	Date														
Immunizations (record dates below)															
DPT															
OPV															
MMR															
Td															
Rubella serology: 11 yr (nonvaccinated female)	Titer														
Tuberculin (tine) test 1, 3, 5, 11, 15 yr	Pos. Neg.														
Hematocrit 1, 5, 13 yr	Result														
Urine culture (female) 5, 8 yr	Nl. Abn.														
Blood pressure 3 yr and each subsequent visit	Result														
Development 6, 18 mo; 3, 5 yr	Nl. Abn. Q.														
Hearing 6 mo; 1, 3 yr; and each subsequent visit	P F														
Vision 4 mo; 1, 3 yr; and each subsequent visit	P F														
Language 2, 3, 5 yr	P F														
Dental care Each visit															
Counseling: each visit															
Nutrition															
Physical care															
Behavior/psychosocial															
Sex education															
Stimulation															
Safety															
Family planning															
Other															

Figure 1-1 Health Maintenance Flow Sheet (1 Week to 17 Years)

discovered, the health maintenance flow sheet is not used for such extra visits.

G. If an indicated procedure is not done or needs to be repeated, the appropriate box of the next assessment is outlined at each visit until the procedure is done. At that time, a check mark is placed in the box or a result is recorded.

H. The information recorded on the health maintenance flow sheet does not have to be recorded in the regular medical record sheet note. The note should contain the interval history, whatever physical examination is done, any medication prescribed, and any details that the provider feels will be helpful for future visits, e.g., certain counseling subjects that will need particular emphasis at future visits.

Note Unlike most health maintenance flow sheets, this one is based on what procedures this particular patient has actually had and what is needed by the specific date of the next scheduled assessment. By merely looking down the column after the date of a scheduled assessment has passed, one can tell what procedures a patient still needs. Thus, audit of health maintenance status is simplified.

III. **Specific procedures**

A. **Assessments** Record the date the patient was seen, the patient's age, and the provider's initials. The 2-week assessment is carried out in the home, and the other visits are in the clinic. Enter the date of the next scheduled assessment in the next column. Note that these are the minimum number of assessments that all patients should have. If problems are discovered, more frequent assessments may be needed. These additional assessments are recorded not on this flow sheet, but in the medical record. A flow sheet for a specific problem, e.g., urinary tract infection, may be indicated.

B. **Complete history** This should be a complete health history, including past medical history, family history, social history, and review of systems. A health questionnaire, which is reviewed with the parent or patient, or both, and commented on in the medical record, is recommended. The history should be taken as soon as possible after registration. The date that it is completed is entered in the appropriate box. At each assessment, an appropriate interval history is taken but need not be noted on the health maintenance flow sheet.

C. **Complete examination** This should be a complete physical examination performed as soon as possible after registration. The date it is completed is entered in the appropriate box. The extent of subse quent physical examinations, which need not be recorded on the flow sheet, is determined by the age-specific health maintenance guidelines (discussed later in this chapter) and by clinical judgment based on the interval medical history and the patient's problem list.

D. **Immunizations**   See Age-Specific Health Maintenance Guidelines (Pediatric) for recommended program. Refer to the *Report of the Committee on Infectious Diseases* (the "Red Book") of the Americ Academy of Pediatrics* for further details. If a patient will need an immunization by the next scheduled assessment, outline the box in next scheduled assessment column and write in the immunization tha will be needed. Place a check mark in the most recently outlined box when immunizations are up to date. A record of the date that each specific immunization is given is entered in the appropriate bo in the Procedures column only and on the immunization record car that is given to parents.

E. **Rubella serology**   If a female 11 years of age or older has not been vaccinated against rubella, her serum rubella antibody titer should b measured. Enter the date and titer.

F. **Tuberculin (tine) test**   Record the date the test is given and the result as positive (pos.) or negative (neg.).

G. **Hematocrit**   Record the date the test is done and the hematocrit value (see Table 1-1).

Table 1-1   Minimum Normal Hematocrit Values at Different Ages

Age	Hematocrit
6 months to 6 years	33
6–14 years	34
Over 14	
(Female)	36
(Male)	40

H. **Urine culture**   Record the date the specimen is collected and the result as normal (Nl.) or abnormal (Abn.). Normal is less than 10,000 organisms per milliliter on a clean midstream specimen. Consult Chapter 9, Urinary Tract (Pediatric), **IV** if the culture has more than 10,000 organisms per milliliter.

*This report is revised and published every few years by the American Academy of Pediatrics, P.O. Box 1034, Evanston, Ill. 60204.

I. **Blood pressure** Record the date and the blood pressure. Be sure to use a cuff that covers two-thirds of the arm, with the inflatable portion completely encircling the arm. Table 1-2 shows normal blood pressure values.

Table 1-2 Maximum Normal Values of Blood Pressure Recorded in the Supine Position

Age (years)	Systolic/Diastolic (mm Hg)
0–3	110/65
3–7	120/70
7–10	130/75
10–13	140/80
13–15	
Male	140/80
Female	140/85
Over 15	140/90

J. **Development** The Denver Developmental Screening Test or a similar, established observational test should be used. Record the date when the test is done. Results are recorded as normal (Nl.), abnormal (Abn.), or questionable (Q.). Although some developmental appraisal should be done at each health maintenance visit, only the result of the formal test is recorded on the flow sheet at the recommended times.

K. **Hearing** Record the date and the result as pass (P) or fail (F). The following screening tests should be used:

1. **Six to 24 months**

   a. Parent gives a history of infant's vocalization and response to sound (see Age-Specific Health Maintenance Guidelines [Pediatric]).

   b. Infant ceases activity on hearing a conversational voice or orients himself toward the voice, or both.

   c. With the infant held, his attention should be fixed on a visual stimulus. The source of sound should be held 4 feet to one side of the infant's head, out of peripheral vision. The infant should respond to low-pitched (clacker or block and hammer), medium-pitched (squeaky toy), and high-pitched (bell) sounds.

2. **Three to 17 years** Pure-tone audiometry. For procedure, see *Standards of Child Health Care* (2nd ed.), Evanston, Ill.: American Academy of Pediatrics, 1972, pp. 127–130.

L. Vision Record the date and the result as pass (P) or fail (F). In ad
tion, record the actual visual acuity in the medical record when the
Snellen E test is used. The following screening tests should be performed:

1. **Under 4 years**

   a. Pupil size, shape, and reaction to light.

   b. Evidence of strabismus by history, position of light reflection
   on cornea, and extraocular movements.

   c. Ability to follow light.

   d. Ability to pick up small, raisin-sized object (over 9 months of
   age).

2. **Four years and over**

   a. Pupil size, shape, and reaction to light.

   b. Evidence of strabismus by history, position of light reflection
   on cornea, and extraocular movements.

   c. Evidence of latent strabismus by cover test.

   d. Snellen E test

      (1) This test is performed with the child placed at a distanc
      of 20 feet from the well-illuminated chart. Each child
      tested on the 20/50, 20/40, 20/30, and 20/20 lines of
      the chart, using both eyes and each alone until the cri-
      teria for failure are met. A child who wears glasses sho
      be tested with and without the glasses. The examiner
      should watch for signs of visual problems such as exces-
      sive blinking, squinting, crossed eyes, or tearing.

      (2) Visual acuity is recorded as the lowest line on the chart
      that is passed. The first number is the distance from th
      testing chart; the second number is the distance at whic
      the particular line of the chart is readable by the norma
      person. Criteria for failure are as follows:

         (a) Failure to read more than half the letters of the
         20/30 line successfully.

         (b) Difference in acuity between eyes of more than c
         line.

         (c) Observation of visual problems by the examiner.

M. **Language** For procedures, see Age-Specific Health Maintenance Guidelines (Pediatric). Record the date and the result as pass (P) or fail (F).

N. **Dental care** Record date. Teeth and gums should be examined and parents and patient counseled on dental care. See Age-Specific Health Maintenance Guidelines (Pediatric) for details. Patients are referred to a dental service for screening and health education at 3 years of age, or at the time of registration if they are older.

O. **Counseling** See Age-Specific Health Maintenance Guidelines (Pediatric) for counseling under each category. Place a check mark in the appropriate box when this has been done.

P. **Other** At the bottom of the flow sheet are empty spaces for other procedures that the provider would like to have as part of an individual's health maintenance program.

AGE-SPECIFIC HEALTH MAINTENANCE GUIDELINES (Pediatric)

Two-Week Home Visit

I. **Provider** Nurse practitioner.

II. **History**

A. Review obstetrical and newborn hospital record.

B. Take interval history.

III. **Examination** Inspection of baby completely undressed.

IV. **Procedures** None.

V. **Dental care**

A. Content of fluoride in drinking water should be 0.7–1.2 ppm.

B. If concentration of fluoride in water or water intake is inadequate, supplemental fluoride should be given, in the form of sodium fluoride (Luride) drops, containing 0.1 mg of fluoride per drop.

1. If water supply has less than 0.3 ppm or baby is breast-fed, give three drops per day.

2. If water supply has 0.4–0.6 ppm and baby consumes some water, give two drops per day.

VI. Counseling

A. Nutrition

1. Discuss breast-feeding:
   a. Breast and nipple care.
   b. Normal balanced diet and good fluid intake for mother.
   c. Feeding technique and schedule.
   d. Misconceptions.
   e. Supplemental vitamins.
   f. Encouragement.
   g. Availability for future counseling if needed.
2. Discuss bottle feeding:
   a. Milk formula selection.
   b. Preparation and storage techniques.
   c. Supplemental vitamins if not in formula.
   d. Feeding technique and schedule.
3. Discuss parents' questions.

B. Physical care

1. Assess adequacy of physical environment for newborn with appropriate counseling or agency referral, or both, as needed.
2. Discuss skin care for baby:
   a. Minor and periodic variations in normal skin.
   b. Bathing techniques.
   c. Care of diaper area.
   d. Care of umbilical cord stump.
   e. Clothing (avoid overheating).
3. Discuss parents' questions.

C. Behavior and psychosocial environment

1. Assess adequacy of emotional environment:

      a. Postpartum depression. Evaluate available supports, e.g., father, grandparents, public health nurse, caretaker, day nursery, social worker.

      b. Mother-infant interaction. Was baby wanted? Is it of the desired sex? What are mother's expectations of baby?

      c. Role of father. Evaluate degree of support he can provide and his expectations of baby.

      d. Adjustment of siblings to baby.

  2. Discuss infant behavior and normal variations:

      a. Crying.

      b. Sleeping and breathing patterns.

      c. Bowel movements.

  3. Assess appropriateness of concepts of discipline and punishment.

  4. Discuss parents' questions.

D. Stimulation (see Infant and Child Stimulation Guidelines, p. 40).

E. Safety

  1. Never leave baby without protection to prevent falling off a surface.

  2. Protect from young siblings.

  3. Protect from pets.

  4. Use special infant seat for automobile. Mother's lap is *not* safe.

F. Family planning.

G. Other areas based on parents' concerns.

VII. Follow-up

A. Explain the purpose of health maintenance visits. Review flow sheet with parents.

B. Give clinic telephone number.

C. Schedule first appointment.

D. Leave medical questionnaire to be completed just before first clinic visit and brought to clinic.

    E. Emphasize availability of health care and counseling before schedul
clinic visit, if needed.

Two-Month Clinic Visit

I. **Provider** Physician.

II. **History**

    A. Review of neonatal hospital summary.

    B. Review of record of 2-week home visit.

    C. Diet.

    D. Development.

    E. Family medical history.

    F. Social history.

    G. Review of systems.

III. **Examination**

    A. Measurements (record on growth chart)

        1. Weight.

        2. Length.

        3. Head circumference.

    B. Complete physical examination.

IV. **Procedures** (immunizations)

    A. Diphtheria-pertussis-tetanus vaccine.

    B. Oral polio vaccine (trivalent).

V. **Dental care** Give supplemental fluoride, if necessary (see Two-Week
Home Visit, **V**).

VI. **Counseling**

    A. Nutrition

        1. Review milk formula or breast-feeding, or both.

        2. Review preparation and storage techniques.

        3. Discuss gradual introduction of solid foods.

        4. Give supplemental vitamins if not in formula or if breast-feeding

5. Discuss iron requirements:

    a. Iron-fortified formula

       or

    b. Ferrous sulfate drops (Fer-In-Sol). For infants weighing 4–7 kg (8–14 lb), give 0.3 ml once a day in water or fruit juice. For infants weighing over 7 kg (over 14 lb) and all premature babies, give 0.6 ml once a day.

6. Discuss parents' questions.

B. Physical care

1. Discuss response of baby to common respiratory and gastrointestinal illnesses, home management, and indications for seeking medical care.

2. Discuss parents' questions.

C. Behavior and psychosocial environment

1. Assess adequacy of emotional environment, with counseling when appropriate:

    a. Maternal-infant interaction: Observe for overprotectiveness, lack of warmth toward baby, signs of maternal depression.

    b. Role of father.

    c. Role of siblings — management of sibling rivalry.

    d. Role of extended family and support system (grandparents, friends).

2. Discuss expected behavior changes before next visit.

3. Discuss parents' questions.

D. Stimulation (see Infant and Child Stimulation Guidelines, p. 40).

E. Safety

1. Never leave baby without protection to prevent falling off a surface.

2. Protect from young siblings.

3. Protect from pets.

4. Prevent contact with objects or toys that are sharp or can be ingested.

      5. Use special infant seat for automobile. Mother's lap is *not* safe.

  F. Family planning.

  G. Other areas based on parents' concerns.

VII. Follow-up   In 2 months, or sooner if necessary.

Four-Month Clinic Visit

  I. Provider   Nurse practitioner.

 II. History   Interval history.

III. Examination

  A. Measurements (record on growth chart)

    1. Weight.

    2. Length.

    3. Head circumference.

  B. Inspection of baby completely undressed.

  C. Extent of further examination: This is based on interval history and patient's problem list.

 IV. Procedures*

  A. Immunizations

    1. Diphtheria-pertussis-tetanus vaccine.

    2. Oral polio vaccine (trivalent).

  B. Developmental appraisal.

  C. Vision screening.

  V. Dental care

  A. Give supplemental fluoride, if necessary (see Two-Week Home Visit V).

  B. Discuss teething and the use of teething toys and hard crackers.

 VI. Counseling

  A. Nutrition

    1. Continue milk formula or breast-feeding, or both.

*See Use of the Health Maintenance Flow Sheet, pp. 4, 5, and 6, for details.

2. Discuss gradual introduction of more solid foods. These can be foods prepared for the family if they are pureed.

3. Give supplemental vitamins if not in formula or if the mother is breast-feeding.

4. Discuss iron requirements:

   a. Iron-fortified formula

   or

   b. Ferrous sulfate drops (Fer-In-Sol). For infants weighing 7 kg or less (14 lb or less), give 0.3 ml once a day in water or fruit juice. For infants weighing over 7 kg (over 14 lb) and all premature babies, give 0.6 ml once a day.

5. Discuss parents' questions.

B. **Physical care**

1. Review response of baby to common respiratory and gastrointestinal illnesses, home management, and indications for seeking medical care.

2. Discuss parents' questions.

C. **Behavior and psychosocial environment**

1. Assess mother-infant interaction and role of father.

2. Discuss alternative caretakers to allow mother time free from baby. Discuss attitude toward mother's returning to work and using day care.

3. Discuss expected behavior changes before next visit.

4. Discuss parents' questions.

D. **Stimulation** (see Infant and Child Stimulation Guidelines, p. 40).

E. **Safety**

1. Discuss baby's increasing mobility and risk of rolling off surface. Keep crib sides up.

2. Protect from young siblings and pets.

3. Prevent contact with objects or toys that are sharp or can be ingested.

4. Do not leave alone in tub of water.

5. Use special infant seat for automobile. Mother's lap is *not* safe.

F. Other areas based on parents' concerns.

VII. **Follow-up**   In 2 months, or sooner if necessary.

Six-Month Clinic Visit

I. **Provider**   Nurse practitioner.

II. **History**   Interval history.

III. **Examination**

A. Measurements (record on growth chart)

1. Weight.

2. Length.

3. Head circumference.

B. Complete physical examination.

IV. **Procedures***

A. Immunizations

1. Diphtheria-pertussis-tetanus vaccine.

2. Oral polio vaccine (trivalent).

B. Developmental appraisal. Perform specific test and record results.

C. Hearing screening. Ask parents the following questions:

1. Does your baby stir or awaken when sleeping quietly and some-one talks or makes a loud noise nearby? (The baby does not have to do this all the time, but should occasionally.)

2. Does your baby sometimes start or jump when there is a very loud noise, such as a cough, dog bark, or object dropped?

V. **Dental care**

A. Give supplemental fluoride, if necessary (see Two-Week Home Visit, V).

B. Discuss teething and the use of teething toys and hard crackers for biting if not done at previous visit.

VI. **Counseling**

*See Use of the Health Maintenance Flow Sheet, pp. 4 and 5, for details.

A. Nutrition

1. Continue milk formula or breast-feeding, or both.

2. Watch for excessive weight gain.

3. Discuss basic food groups and avoidance of nonnutritious sugared commercial foods.

4. Discuss need for supplemental vitamins if not in formula or if breast-feeding.

5. Discuss iron requirements:

   a. Iron-fortified formula

      or

   b. Ferrous sulfate drops (Fer-In-Sol), 0.6 ml once a day in water or fruit juice

      and

   c. Iron-containing foods.

6. Discuss parents' questions.

B. Physical care

1. Review parental management of illnesses occurring since previous visit.

2. Discuss parents' questions.

C. Behavior and psychosocial environment

1. Assess maternal-infant interaction and role of father.

2. Discuss parents' attitude toward discipline. Emphasize that the baby is too young to "behave."

3. Discuss adjustment of siblings to baby.

4. Discuss stranger anxiety — baby-sitter should be familiar to the baby before parents leave.

5. Discuss parents' questions.

D. Stimulation (see Infant and Child Stimulation Guidelines, p. 41).

E. Safety

1. Discuss baby's increasing mobility and risk of falling off a surface.

   2. Protect from young siblings and pets.

   3. Prevent contact with objects or toys that are sharp or can be ingested, especially those that can be reached while the child is crawling.

   4. Do not leave alone in tub of water.

   5. Use special infant seat for automobile. Mother's lap is *not* safe while riding in a car.

F. **Other areas based on parents' concerns.**

VII. **Follow-up**   In 3 months, or sooner if necessary.

Nine-Month Clinic Visit

  I. **Provider**   Nurse practitioner.

 II. **History**   Interval history.

III. **Examination**

   A. Measurements (record on growth chart)

   1. Weight.

   2. Length.

   3. Head circumference.

   B. Inspection of baby completely undressed.

   C. Extent of further examination: This is based on interval history and patient's problem list.

 IV. **Procedures**

   A. Review of flow sheet to be certain procedures indicated at previous visits have been completed.

   B. Developmental appraisal.

  V. **Dental care**

   A. Examine teeth.

   B. Give supplemental fluoride, if necessary (see Two-Week Home Visit, V).

   C. To prevent caries, eliminate all beverages except plain water from a nursing bottle that is left in the crib with the baby.

   D. Clean teeth with gauze pad once a day.

VI. Counseling

A. Nutrition

1. Continue milk formula or breast-feeding, or both.

2. Review diet. Counsel on importance of basic food groups and avoidance of nonnutritious sugared commercial foods. Consider family preferences and economic factors.

3. Give supplemental vitamins if not in formula or if breast-feeding.

4. Discuss iron requirements:

    a. Iron-fortified formula

       or

    b. Ferrous sulfate drops (Fer-In-Sol), 0.6 ml once a day in water or fruit juice

       and

    c. Iron-containing foods.

5. Discuss management of food preferences and possible decrease in appetite.

B. Physical care

1. Review parental management of illnesses occurring since previous visit.

2. Discuss parents' questions.

C. Behavior and psychosocial environment

1. Assess family's response to annoying behavior. Help parents to realize that baby is not yet able to be disciplined.

2. Discuss stranger and separation anxiety.

3. Discuss child's desire to use spoon and cup for feeding and expected messiness.

4. Discuss parents' questions and expectations of baby.

D. Stimulation (see Infant and Child Stimulation Guidelines, p. 41).

E. Safety

1. Prepare home for increasing mobility:

    a. Cover electric outlets with plug guards.

      b. Disconnect all cords to appliances when not in use.

      c. Take objects out of reach, off floor and low tables.

      d. Remove sharp or small objects from sight and reach.

      e. Lock medicines, cleaning materials, and poisons away and out of reach, and prescribe and discuss the use of syrup of ipecac (see Chapter 2, Ingestions and Poisonings [Pediatric], **VI. E).**

      f. Keep handles of pots, etc., turned away from reach.

      g. Keep hot food containers out of reach on tables.

      h. Put gate across top of stairs.

      i. Place guards in front of space heaters, heating stoves, and radiators.

      j. Keep screens in open windows.

   2. Use special infant seat for automobile. Mother's lap is *not* safe.

   3. Do not leave alone in tub or near pool.

   4. Keep child in enclosed space when outside and not in company of adult.

  F. Other areas based on parents' questions.

VII. Follow-up   In 3 months, or sooner if necessary.

Twelve-Month Clinic Visit

  I. Provider   Physician.

 II. History   Interval history.

III. Examination

  A. Measurements (record on growth chart)

    1. Weight.

    2. Length.

    3. Head circumference.

  B. Complete physical examination.

IV. Procedures*

  A. Immunization: Measles-mumps-rubella vaccine.

*See Use of the Health Maintenance Flow Sheet, pp. 4, 5, and 6, for details.

   B. Tuberculin skin test.

   C. Hematocrit determination (normal is greater than 32%).

   D. Developmental appraisal.

   E. Hearing screening. Ask parents the following questions:

   1. Does your baby turn his head in any direction to find an interesting sound or the person speaking?

   2. Does your baby stir or awaken when sleeping quietly and someone talks or makes a loud sound nearby?

   F. Vision screening.

V. **Dental care**

   A. Examine teeth.

   B. Give supplemental fluoride, if necessary (see Two-Week Home Visit, V).

   C. To prevent caries, eliminate all beverages except plain water from nursing bottles, if still drinking from a bottle.

   D. Discourage frequent snacking of sugar-containing foods by child.

   E. Clean teeth with soft toothbrush or gauze pad once a day.

VI. **Counseling**

   A. Nutrition

   1. Try to keep milk intake under 20 ounces if a balanced diet is available.

   2. Review diet. Counsel again, if necessary, on importance of basic food groups and avoidance of nonnutritious sugared commercial foods. Consider family preferences and economic factors.

   3. Continue iron-fortified formula *or* ferrous sulfate drops (Fer-In-Sol), 0.6 ml once a day in water or juice.

   4. If necessary, discuss again management of food preferences and possible decrease in appetite.

   B. Physical care

   1. Review parental management of illnesses occurring since previous visit.

   2. Discuss parents' questions.

C. **Behavior and psychosocial environment**

   1. Discuss parents' concept of acceptable behavior and discipline and their expectations.

   2. Discuss adjustment of family to curiosity, mobility, and negativism of baby and their tolerance of noise from baby and siblings.

   3. Discuss management of separations.

   4. Explore parents' concept of toilet training.

   5. Discuss progress of child toward drinking mainly from cup.

   6. Discuss parents' questions.

D. **Stimulation** (see Infant and Child Stimulation Guidelines, p. 42).

E. **Safety** (see Nine-Month Clinic Visit, **VI.E**).

F. **Other areas based on parents' questions.**

VII. **Follow-up**   In 6 months, or sooner if necessary.

Eighteen-Month Clinic Visit

I. **Provider**   Nurse practitioner.

II. **History**

A. Interval history.

B. Review and revision of family and social history.

III. **Examination**

A. Measurements (record on growth chart)

   1. Weight.

   2. Length.

   3. Head circumference.

B. Inspection of baby completely undressed.

C. Extent of further examination: This is based on interval history and patient's problem list.

IV. **Procedures***

A. Immunizations

   1. Diphtheria-pertussis-tetanus vaccine.

*See Use of the Health Maintenance Flow Sheet, pp. 4 and 5, for details.

     2. Oral polio vaccine (trivalent).

   B. Developmental appraisal. Perform specific test and record results.

V. **Dental care**

   A. Examine teeth.

   B. Give supplemental fluoride, if necessary (see Two-Week Home Visit, **V**).

   C. Discourage frequent snacking of sugar-containing foods by child.

   D. Clean teeth with soft toothbrush or gauze pad twice a day.

VI. **Counseling**

   A. **Nutrition**

     1. Review diet. Counsel again, if necessary, on importance of basic food groups and avoidance of nonnutritious sugared commercial foods. Consider family preferences and economic factors.

     2. Limit milk intake to 2 or 3 glasses per day if a balanced diet is available.

     3. Discuss progress of self-feeding.

     4. Discuss parents' questions.

   B. **Physical care**

     1. Review parental management of illnesses occurring since previous visit.

     2. Discuss parents' questions.

   C. **Behavior and psychosocial environment**

     1. Discuss adjustment of family to baby's negativism, and possible frustration of parents' expectations of baby.

     2. Discuss discipline and limit setting. Encourage parents to use substitution and positive reinforcement rather than physical punishment.

     3. Management of separation from mother.

     4. Discuss toilet training and variations in normal patterns.

     5. Discuss sleep problems, e.g., night terrors, desire to sleep in parents' room.

     6. Discuss parents' questions.

    D. Stimulation (see Infant and Child Stimulation Guidelines, p. 42).

    E. Safety Review hazards and precautions discussed at previous visit (see Nine-Month Clinic Visit, **VI.E**).

    F. Other areas based on parents' questions.

VII. Follow-up In 6 months, or sooner if necessary.

Two-Year Clinic Visit

  I. Provider Nurse practitioner.

 II. History Interval history.

III. Examination

    A. Measurements (record on growth chart)

       1. Weight.

       2. Length.

       3. Head circumference.

    B. Complete physical examination.

IV. Procedures*

    A. Developmental appraisal.

    B. Hearing screening

       1. Does baby point to at least one part of the body (eyes, feet, etc.) when you ask, without seeing your lips?

       2. Does baby point to the right picture when asked, "Where's the cat [or dog, man, horse, etc.]?" without seeing your lips?

       3. Does baby give you a toy or put an object on a table or chair when you ask, without seeing your lips?

    Note Baby may pass by observation of examiner or report of parent. Since this test evaluates more than just hearing function, failure requires further evaluation of other aspects of development as well.

    C. **Language screening** Ask parent what words the child uses regularly to denote specific objects, persons, or actions. This procedure is passed if parent reports child has three words other than *da-da* or *ma-ma*. Words do not have to be intelligible, but they must be specific.

*See Use of the Health Maintenance Flow Sheet, p. 5, for details.

V. Dental care

A. Examine teeth.

B. Give supplemental fluoride, if necessary:

  1. Content of fluoride in drinking water should be 0.7–1.2 ppm.

  2. If concentration in water or water intake is inadequate, sodium fluoride (Luride) drops, containing 0.1 mg of fluoride per drop should be given:

   a. If water supply has less than 0.3 ppm, give 5 drops per day.

   b. If water supply has 0.4–0.6 ppm, give 3 drops per day.

C. Discuss rationale for avoiding frequent snacking of sugar-containing foods.

D. Remind parents to clean teeth with toothbrush or gauze pad twice a day.

E. Refer to dental services before age 3 even if teeth appear normal.

VI. Counseling

A. Nutrition

  1. Review diet. Counsel again, if necessary, on importance of basic food groups, avoidance of nonnutritious sugared commercial foods, and limiting of milk to 2 or 3 glasses per day if a balanced diet is available. Consider family preferences and economic factors.

  2. Discuss progress of self-feeding.

  3. Discuss parents' questions.

B. Physical care

  1. Review parental management of illnesses occurring since previous visit.

  2. Discuss parents' questions.

C. Behavior and psychosocial environment

  1. Discuss parents' concepts of normal behavior and limits. Discuss the fact that child understands no before inner controls are available to obey.

  2. Discuss discipline and use of substitution and positive reinforcement instead of physical punishment.

     3. Discuss beginning of toilet training. Encourage independence in toileting when day control is achieved.

     4. Management of separation from mother.

     5. Discuss sleep problems.

     6. Discuss parents' questions.

  D. Stimulation (see Infant and Child Stimulation Guidelines, p. 42).

  E. Safety

     1. Lock doors where danger of falling exists (e.g., cellar).

     2. Lock up sharp or electrical tools.

     3. Check driveway, while outside automobile, before backing up.

     4. Lock all car doors.

     5. Never leave child unrestrained in cargo section of station wagon.

     6. Put matches out of reach.

     7. See also Nine-Month Clinic Visit, **VI.E.**

VII. Follow-up   In 1 year, or sooner if necessary.

Three-Year Clinic Visit

  I. Provider   Nurse practitioner.

 II. History

  A. Interval history.

  B. Review and revision of family and social history.

III. Examination

  A. Measurements (record on growth chart)

     1. Weight.

     2. Length.

  B. Complete physical examination.

IV. Procedures*

  A. Tuberculin skin test.

  B. Blood pressure (normal is less than 120/70 mm Hg in the supine po

*See Use of the Health Maintenance Flow Sheet, pp. 4, 5, and 6, for details.

    C. Developmental appraisal. Perform specific test and record results.

    D. Hearing screening.

    E. Vision screening.

    F. Language screening. This test is passed if child makes sentences of three or more words and speech is largely intelligible to strangers.

V. Dental care

    A. Examine teeth.

    B. Give supplemental fluoride, if necessary (see Two-Year Clinic Visit, V.B).

    C. Discuss rationale for avoiding frequent snacking of sugar-containing foods.

    D. Remind parents to brush child's teeth twice a day with anticariogenic toothpaste.

    E. Refer if patient was not seen by dental service within the previous year.

VI. Counseling

A. Nutrition

    1. Review diet. Counsel again, if necessary, on importance of basic food groups and avoidance of nonnutritious sugared commercial foods. Consider family preferences and economic factors.

    2. Discuss possibility of periods of decreased appetite.

    3. Explain that eating patterns are influenced by other members of family.

    4. Discuss parents' questions.

B. Physical care

    1. Review parental management of illnesses occurring since previous visit.

    2. Discuss parents' questions.

C. Behavior and psychosocial environment

    1. Discuss balance between need for independence and realistic discipline, guidance, and limits.

    2. Discuss need for social interaction with peers.

3. Discuss normal early childhood fears (e.g., bodily injury), imagination (which is different from lying), and curiosity.

4. Discuss value and characteristics of good nursery school and day care. Assist family in identifying a program, if desired.

5. Discuss sibling rivalry if new baby is due or has arrived.

6. Discuss normal lapses in bladder and bowel control. Issue is not to be made of these with child.

7. Discuss parents' questions.

D. **Sex education** (age 3–5 years)

1. Explore parents' concept of normal psychosexual development in preschool child.

2. Discuss sexual identity and common questions asked by children, including masturbation and sexual curiosity about other children's anatomy.

E. **Stimulation** (see Infant and Child Stimulation Guidelines, p. 45).

F. **Safety**

1. Lock doors where danger of falling exists (e.g., cellar).

2. Place screens or guards over windows.

3. Place guards in front of all space heaters, heating stoves, and radiators.

4. Lock up sharp or electrical tools and firearms.

5. Lock up poisons and medications. Review use of syrup of ipecac (see Chapter 2, Ingestions and Poisonings [Pediatric], **VI.E**).

6. Teach child to watch out for moving automobiles in driveways and streets.

7. Use special young child's car seat for automobile. Shoulder belt may be used. Never leave child unrestrained in cargo section of station wagon.

8. Lock all car doors.

9. Never allow child to swim or wade in water unsupervised by adult.

G. Other areas based on parents' questions.

VII. **Follow-up**   In 2 years, or sooner if necessary.

Five-Year Clinic Visit

I. Provider   Nurse practitioner.

II. History

    A. Interval history, including complete review of systems.

    B. Review and revision of family and social history.

III. Examination

    A. Measurements (record on growth chart)

        1. Weight.

        2. Length.

    B. Complete physical examination.

IV. Procedures*

    A. Immunizations

        1. Administer diphtheria-pertussis-tetanus vaccine.

        2. Give oral polio vaccine (trivalent).

        3. Be certain child has had measles-mumps-rubella vaccine.

    B. Tuberculin skin test.

    C. Hematocrit determination (normal is 33% or greater).

    D. Urine culture (girls only).

    E. Blood pressure (normal is less than 120/70 mm Hg in the supine position.

    F. Developmental appraisal. Perform specific test and record the results.

    G. Hearing screening.

    H. Vision screening.

    I. Language screening. This test is failed if child does any of the following:

        1. Often substitutes easy for difficult sounds, e.g., *wabbit.*

        2. Constantly drops word endings.

        3. Stutters or stammers.

*See Use of the Health Maintenance Flow Sheet, pp. 4, 5, and 6, for details.

      4. Speaks in a monotonous voice.

      5. Speaks in a voice that is excessively loud or inaudible.

      6. Speaks with hypernasality or hyponasality.

V. Dental care

A. Examine teeth.

B. If water supply has less than 0.7 ppm of fluoride, prescribe 1 tablet per day of sodium fluoride (Luride Lozi-Tabs, which releases 1 mg of fluoride per tablet).

C. Discuss rationale for avoiding frequent snacking of sugar-containing foods.

D. Remind patient to brush teeth twice a day with anticariogenic tooth paste.

E. Refer if patient was not seen by dental service within previous year.

VI. Counseling (age 5–8 years)

A. Nutrition

1. Discuss parents' anxieties about eating problems. Encourage child's independence, i.e., have nutritious foods available but allow child to choose amount and kind of food for his own plate. Reassure parents with growth chart if they are concerned about adequate intake.

2. Emphasize importance of breakfast, especially when child is going to school all day.

3. Discuss nutritious after-school snacks.

4. Encourage parents not to focus on *strict* table manners. Mealtime should be enjoyable for family.

5. Discuss parents' questions.

B. Physical care

1. Review parental management of illnesses occurring since previous visit.

2. Discuss importance of adequate sleep and consistent sleep routine

3. Discuss teaching child personal hygiene.

4. Discuss parents' questions.

C. **Behavior and psychosocial environment**

1. Discuss preparing child for separation and independence associated with attending school. Assess parental concerns.

2. Discuss importance of regular school attendance.

3. Discuss importance of parent-teacher relationship and periodic meetings.

4. Discuss importance of peer acceptance and need for praise.

5. Discuss the worries and fears common in early school-age children, e.g., death, competition with peers, parental marital conflict, need to achieve. Discuss signs of excessive stress and availability of health provider for counseling, if needed.

6. Discuss parents' expectations of child, e.g., chores, self-discipline, handling of anger. Are they realistic?

7. Discuss potential problems with teacher after obtaining parental permission.

D. **Sex education**

1. Explore parents' preparedness for potential questions.

2. Encourage parents to be aware of the scope of sex education programs in school.

E. **Stimulation**   Parents should be encouraged to do the following:

1. Converse with child regularly. Listen to child and encourage expression of thoughts.

2. Read to child and have child read to them.

3. Be sure child can dress completely.

4. Provide pencil, crayons, paper, paints, and scissors.

5. Show interest in child's schoolwork and provide encouragement.

6. Teach child responsible use of money.

7. Review television viewing habits. Encourage balanced selective viewing of educational and entertaining programs.

F. **Safety**   Parents should be encouraged to do the following:

1. Teach child to watch for moving automobiles, especially at intersections. Teach traffic signals and rules.

2. Teach bicycle techniques, traffic rules for bicycles, and danger from automobiles.

3. Teach child swimming skills. Never allow child to swim unsupervised by adult.

4. Discuss fire prevention in the home with the child.

5. Lock up firearms.

6. Do not allow dangerous tools to be used unsupervised.

7. Have child and entire family use seat and shoulder belts for automobile safety. Lock all car doors. Do not allow child to ride in cargo section of station wagon.

G. Other areas based on parents' questions.

VII. **Follow-up**   In 3 years, or sooner if necessary.

Eight-Year Clinic Visit

I. **Provider**   Nurse practitioner.

II. **History**

A. Interval history, including complete review of systems.

B. Review and revision of family and social history.

III. **Examination**

A. Measurements (record on growth chart)

1. Weight.

2. Height.

B. Complete physical examination.

IV. **Procedures***

A. Urine culture (girls only).

B. Blood pressure (normal is less than 130/75 mm Hg in the supine position).

C. Hearing screening.

D. Vision screening.

*See Use of the Health Maintenance Flow Sheet, pp. 4, 5, and 6, for details.

V. **Dental care**

  A. Examine teeth.

  B. Give supplemental fluoride, if necessary (see Five-Year Clinic Visit, **V.B**).

  C. Discuss rationale for avoiding frequent snacking of sugar-containing foods.

  D. Remind patient to brush teeth twice a day with anticariogenic toothpaste and floss once a day.

  E. Refer if patient was not seen by dental service within previous year.

VI. **Counseling** (age 8–11 years)

  A. **Nutrition**

   1. Review diet. Counsel again, if necessary, on importance of basic food groups and avoidance of nonnutritious sugared commercial foods. Consider family preferences and economic factors.

   2. Emphasize importance of breakfast, especially when child is going to school all day.

   3. Discuss nutritious after-school snacks.

   4. Discuss parents' questions.

  B. **Physical care**

   1. Review parental management of illnesses occurring since previous visit.

   2. Discuss importance of adequate sleep.

   3. Discuss parents' questions.

  C. **Behavior and psychosocial environment**

   1. Discuss school adjustment and progress with child and parents.

   2. Discuss problems with teacher after obtaining parental permission.

   3. Discuss importance of parent-teacher relationship and periodic meetings.

   4. Explore peer relationships and involvement in group activities, e.g., scouts, religious groups, summer camp, summer recreational programs.

5. Discuss child's interpersonal relationships with siblings and with parents.

6. Discuss parents' and child's attitudes toward responsibilities, e.g. chores, neatness, monetary allowance.

7. Pursue child's as well as parents' concerns.

D. **Sex education**

1. Discuss parents' response to questions raised by child since previous visit.

2. Encourage parents to be aware of the scope of sex education program in school and to complement it as appropriate.

3. Discuss possibility of menarche before next visit and parents' plans for discussion with daughter.

4. Discuss parents' concerns.

E. **Stimulation**   Parents should be encouraged to do the following:

1. Converse with child regularly. Listen to child and encourage expression of thoughts.

2. Show interest in child's schoolwork.

3. Provide child with quiet area with as much privacy as possible.

4. Encourage application of skills learned at school, including the following:

   a. Reading: Encourage use of library.

   b. Mathematics: Assist child in planning use of money.

   c. Art, music, woodworking: Provide child with simple equipment as desired.

5. Review television-viewing habits. Encourage balanced selective viewing of educational and entertaining programs.

F. **Safety**   Parents should be encouraged to do the following:

1. Teach child the rules of pedestrian and cycling safety.

2. Encourage development of swimming, water, and boating safety skills. Never allow child to swim unsupervised by older person.

3. Discuss fire prevention in home and use of telephone for emergencies.

      4. Lock up firearms.

      5. Do not allow electrical tools to be used unsupervised.

      6. Have child and entire family use seat and shoulder belts for automobile safety. Lock all car doors.

    G. Other areas based on parents' questions.

VII. **Follow-up** In 3 years, or sooner if necessary.

Eleven-Year Clinic Visit

  I. **Provider** Nurse practitioner.

 II. **History**

    A. Interval history, including complete review of systems.

    B. Review and revision of family and social history.

III. **Examination**

    A. Measurements (record on growth chart)

      1. Weight.

      2. Height.

    B. Complete physical examination.

IV. **Procedures***

    A. Rubella serology (nonvaccinated females).

    B. Tuberculin skin test.

    C. Blood pressure (normal is less than 140/80 mm Hg in the supine position).

    D. Hearing screening.

    E. Vision screening.

 V. **Dental care**

    A. Examine teeth.

    B. Give supplemental fluoride, if necessary (see Five-Year Clinic Visit, V.B).

    C. Discuss rationale for avoiding frequent snacks of sugar-containing foods.

*See Use of the Health Maintenance Flow Sheet, pp. 4, 5, and 6, for details.

D. Remind patient to brush teeth twice a day with anticariogenic tooth paste and floss once a day.

E. Refer if patient was not seen by dental service within previous year.

VI. Counseling

A. Nutrition

1. Review diet. Counsel parents and child, if necessary, on importance of basic food groups and avoidance of nonnutritious sugared commercial goods. Consider family preferences and economic factors.

2. Emphasize importance of breakfast, especially when child is going to school all day.

3. Discuss nutritious after-school snacks.

4. Discuss parents' and child's questions.

B. Physical care

1. Review parental management of illnesses since previous visit.

2. Discuss importance of adequate sleep and exercise.

3. Discuss with patient physical changes associated with puberty and the wide variation in time of onset.

4. Discuss skin care relative to acne.

5. Discuss parents' and child's questions.

C. Behavior and psychosocial environment

1. Discuss school adjustment and progress with child and parents. Assess degree of parental involvement and concern.

2. Discuss problems with school personnel after obtaining parental permission.

3. Discuss importance of parent-teacher relationship and periodic meetings.

4. Discuss attitudes of parents and child toward school, achievement and long-range plans. Are they realistic?

5. Explore peer relationships and involvement in group activities, e.g., scouts, YMCA or YWCA, religious groups, summer camp, summer recreational programs.

6. Discuss with parents normal increased desire for independence combined with need for consistent limits and someone who will *listen* to child's concerns.

7. Discuss child's interpersonal relationships with siblings and parents.

8. Discuss parents' and child's attitudes toward responsibilities, e.g., chores, neatness, monetary allowance.

9. Pursue child's and parents' concerns.

D. Sex education

1. Discuss parents' response to questions raised by child since previous visit.

2. Discuss child's understanding of menarche and parents' plans for discussion with daughter.

3. Discuss variable increase in interest in opposite sex.

4. Discuss with parents the normal child's concerns and need for sex education, especially, girls who mature early. Counsel patient as needed and desired by parents in mechanism of pregnancy and high-risk relationships. Plan another visit for counseling in this area before next health maintenance visit (age 13), if appropriate. Emphasize to patient and parents your availability.

E. Safety Parents should be encouraged to do the following:

1. Reinforce the rules of pedestrian and cycling safety.

2. Encourage development of swimming, water, and boating safety skills. Never allow child to swim alone.

3. Discuss fire prevention in the home and use of telephone for emergencies.

4. If firearms are available, instruct child in safe use.

5. Have child and entire family use seat and shoulder belts for automobile safety. Lock all car doors.

F. Other areas based on parents' questions.

VII. Follow-up In 2 years, or sooner as needed.

Thirteen- and 15-Year Clinic Visit

I. Provider Nurse practitioner.

II. History

A. Interval history, including complete review of systems.

B. Review and revision of family and social history.

III. Examination

A. Measurements (record on growth chart)

1. Weight.

2. Height.

B. Complete physical examination.

IV. Procedures*

A. Immunization: Tetanus-diphtheria toxoid (adult type-Td), if 10 years have elapsed since previous booster.

B. Tuberculin skin test at age 15.

C. Hematocrit determination at age 13 (normal is greater than 33%).

D. Blood pressure (normal is less than 140/80 mm Hg for males and less than 140/85 mm Hg for females in the supine position).

E. Hearing screening.

F. Vision screening.

V. Dental care

A. Examine teeth.

B. Discuss rationale for avoiding frequent snacks of sugar-containing foods.

C. Remind patient to brush teeth twice a day with anticariogenic tooth paste and floss once a day.

D. Refer if patient was not seen by dental service within previous year

VI. Counseling (age 13–15 years). Nurse practitioner should meet separately with patient and parents.

A. Nutrition

1. Review diet. Counsel patient and parents again, if necessary, on importance of basic food groups. Consider family preferences and economic factors.

*See Use of the Health Maintenance Flow Sheet, pp. 4, 5, and 6, for details.

   2. Emphasize importance of breakfast, especially when patient is going to school all day.

   3. Discuss nutritious after-school snacks.

   4. Discuss patient's and parents' questions.

B. **Physical care**

   1. Review home management of illnesses occurring since previous visit.

   2. Discuss importance of adequate sleep and exercise.

   3. Discuss patient's and parents' questions about physical changes associated with puberty.

   4. Discuss skin care relative to acne.

   5. Discuss patient's and parents' questions.

C. **Behavior and psychosocial environment**

   1. Discuss school adjustment and progress with patient and parents.

   2. Discuss problems with school personnel after obtaining permission.

   3. Emphasize practical importance of school relative to careers and employment, if necessary.

   4. Explore peer relationships and involvement in group activities.

   5. Discuss with parents how to achieve a balance between adolescent's appropriate desire for independence and need for consistent, fair limits and someone who will *listen* to concerns.

   6. Discuss with patient and parents interpersonal relationships with siblings and parents (individually, or joint conference if desired by patient).

   7. Discuss with parents the adolescent's need for occasional privacy.

   8. Discuss with patient concerns about body image and being different, e.g., acne, tallness, fatness, shortness, delayed puberty.

   9. Assess and discuss patient's and parents' attitudes toward alcohol, smoking, and drugs. Counsel as appropriate.

D. **Sex education**   Extent of counseling at a particular visit will depend on maturity, experience, and stage of development of patient. Special visits with teenager for counseling in this area should be scheduled at appropriate times during adolescence.

1. Discuss patient's relationship with opposite sex and his or her concerns.

2. Assess patient's understanding of anatomy and physiology of reproduction.

3. Assess the immediacy of patient's need for contraceptive information and specific management. Discuss with patient the approach to be taken with parents.

4. Discuss with patient the responsibility that both male and femal have for sexual activity and contraception.

5. Discuss venereal disease.

6. Discuss patient's and parents' questions.

E. **Safety**   Encourage the following:

1. Enrollment in driver-education course.

2. Use of seat and shoulder belts for automobile safety.

3. Development of swimming, water, and boating safety skills. Ne swim alone.

4. Safe use of firearms, if these are available.

F. Other areas based on patient's and parents' questions.

VII. **Follow-up**   In 2 years, or sooner as needed.

Seventeen-Year Clinic Visit

I. **Provider**   Nurse practitioner.

II. **History**

A. Interval history, including complete review of systems.

B. Review and revision of family and social history.

III. **Examination**

A. Measurements

1. Weight.

2. Height.

B. Complete physical examination.

IV. **Procedures***

*See Use of the Health Maintenance Flow Sheet, pp. 4, 5, and 6, for details.

A. Immunization: Tetanus-diphtheria toxoid (adult type-Td), if 10 years have elapsed since previous booster.

B. Blood pressure (normal is less than 140/90 mm Hg in the supine position).

C. Hearing screening.

D. Vision screening.

V. Dental care

A. Examine teeth.

B. Discuss rationale for avoiding frequent snacks of sugar-containing foods.

C. Remind patient to brush teeth twice a day and floss once a day.

D. Refer if patient was not seen by dental service within the previous year.

VI. Counseling

A. Nutrition

1. Review diet. Counsel on importance of basic food groups. Consider family preferences and economic factors.

2. Emphasize importance of breakfast.

B. Physical care

1. Review home management of illnesses occurring since previous visit.

2. Discuss importance of adequate sleep and regular exercise.

3. Discuss patient's questions.

C. Behavior and psychosocial environment

1. Discuss school adjustment and progress.

2. Discuss future career and education plans.

3. Discuss relationship with opposite sex and his or her concerns.

4. Discuss interpersonal relationship with parents (individual interview, and joint conference with parents if desired by patient).

5. Assess and discuss patient's attitudes toward alcohol, smoking, and drugs. Counsel as appropriate.

D. **Sex education**

1. Discuss patient's concerns about relationship with opposite sex.

2. Discuss contraception and responsibility of both male and femal

3. Discuss venereal disease.

E. **Safety**   Encourage the following:

1. Discuss enrollment in driver-education course. If patient is alrea driving, emphasize the great risk of injury and death associated with poor driving habits. Review the association of alcohol with automobile accidents.

2. Discuss use of seat and shoulder belts for automobile safety. Review statistics establishing their value.

3. Discuss development of swimming, water, and boating safety sk Emphasize that one should never swim alone.

F. Other areas based on patient's questions.

VII. **Follow-up**   In 3 years, or sooner if needed. If provider does not care adults, arrange referral at this visit.

INFANT AND CHILD STIMULATION GUIDELINES

Birth to 6 Months

I. **Language and personal-social development**

A. Talk and sing to the baby even though he cannot understand what you say.

B. Repeat the noises he makes.

C. While he is awake, place him where he can see and hear what is going on.

II. **Visual, auditory, and tactile stimulation**

A. **Hang pictures on the wall or crib** where the baby can see them. Cu pictures from magazines or use pictures that older children bring home from school.

B. **Hang dangling toys above the baby:**

1. Attach ribbon, bright cloth, colored paper, ball, shiny spoon, painted spools, measuring spoons, rubber jar rings, etc., to a string or coat hanger and hang it across the crib.

2. Make a mobile. Cut a circle from cardboard or a plastic bleach bottle. Using thread, tie on colorful cutouts from boxes (e.g., circles, birds, butterflies). Hang the mobile from a light fixture or the ceiling over the crib.

C. **Make rattles (noisemakers)** Fill small cardboard boxes, plastic salt shakers, soft drink cans, etc., with large stones, bottle caps, poker chips, large buttons, spools, etc., and tape the end shut. (Use large objects that he cannot swallow just in case the rattle comes apart.)

D. **Make soft, cuddly toys** Sew two pieces of cloth (old towel, cut in pattern) together and stuff with rags, nylons, cotton batting, facial tissues, or toilet paper, or stuff an old sock or glove.

E. **Put the child on a blanket on the floor** Let baby see more of the world around him and have an opportunity to exercise his muscles.

Six to 12 Months

I. **Language and personal-social development**

A. **Talk to him** — tell him what you are doing to or with him even though he does not understand.

B. **Point to objects and people** and name them over and over.

C. **Play games** with him (e.g., patty cake, peek-a-boo, where is Johnny's nose?, etc.).

D. While he is awake, **have him in the room with you.** Let him crawl on the floor and explore or put him in a walker.

E. **Let him see himself in the mirror** Talk to him while he is looking in the mirror — "Look at baby's nose," "Here is Johnny's mouth."

II. **Visual, auditory, and tactile stimulation**

A. **Provide soft, cuddly toys.**

B. **Make noisemakers:**

1. Make a drum out of an empty oatmeal box and give the child a stick with which to bang on it.

2. Fill containers of different shapes with previously mentioned articles (see Birth to 6 Months, **II.C**).

C. **Give him objects to handle and explore** (objects that are unbreakable and too large to be swallowed). When the child is in his walker, tie these objects to the walker so that he can handle and play with them.

1. Let him play with a rolling pin, large spoons, boxes (cereal, shoe, berry, match), bowls, pots, pans, cans, baking tins (cake, pie, muffin), plastic cups, screw-top plastic bottles, coffee pot, bandage cans, etc.

2. Present a variety of textures (hard, soft, fuzzy, smooth, etc.), sponges, different types of material (velvet, imitation fur, cotton, wool) by making a ball out of different textured materials and stuffing it with cotton, rags, nylons, etc.

D. **Provide fill'-n'-dump toys**   Use a container with a large opening (e.g., milk carton, coffee can, oatmeal box) and small objects to place in the container and dump out (e.g., spools, measuring spoons, clothes pins, corks, poker chips).

E. **Put baby's favorite toy in a paper bag** and have him find it.

One to 3 Years

I. **Language development**

A. **Talk to the child** — listen with interest to what he has to say. Use complete thoughts — not "Pick it up," but "Pick up the ball from under the table."

B. **Read to him** or tell him stories.

C. **Have him tell you stories** about pictures in books or magazines. **Make a picture book.** Cut out large pieces of paper bag for the cover and pages. Fold them in half and tie them together with string or yarn. Paste pictures in the book from magazines, cereal boxes, newspapers, etc.

D. **Name parts of his body** and pictures of people. Have him name objects.

E. **Let him look in a mirror** and point out his facial features and body parts.

F. **Play singing games** (e.g., "Ring Around the Rosy," "Row, Row, Row Your Boat," "Three Blind Mice").

G. **Play telephone** with him.

H. **Play with puppets**; have a conversation using puppets.

1. **Paper bag puppets**   Fill the end of a small bag with cotton or crumpled newspaper, insert a stick or pencil, tie a string around the stuffed area and stick-paint, draw, or color a face on the bag.

    2. Potato puppets   Insert a stick in a small potato. Facial features can be created by painting the surface of the potato or using bits of paper held in place with pins.

    3. Potato finger puppets   Make by cutting a small hole in the bottom of the potato and slipping the potato over one's finger.

    4. Old-glove puppets   Cut off the fingers and thumb and stuff them with cotton, nylons, old rags, etc. The thumb becomes the head and body of the puppet, two fingers become the arms when sewn to the thumb section. Bind the head and waist sections off with string or yarn. Decorate with pieces of material, yarn, and ribbon.

II. Personal-social development

  A. Let the child play with **dolls and stuffed animals.**

  B. Take him to the store, to a neighbor's house, riding in car, on the bus, to the park and zoo. Point to and name people, objects, and animals.

  C. Play **games** such as hide and seek with him.

  D. Allow the child to experiment with dressing up and with **adult role playing.**

    1. Give the child mother's or father's old hats, dresses, suits, shoes, purses, and wallets.

    2. Make hats and masks out of paper bags or paper plates. Make dresses out of blankets or material.

    3. Let the child use cooking utensils, house-cleaning equipment, and safe tools.

    4. Make a house by putting a blanket over a high table.

III. Gross motor development

  A. Push-pull toys

    1. Attach a string to a large box and fill it with light-weight objects.

    2. Make a train by tying boxes (shoe boxes, milk cartons, salt boxes, etc.) together with heavy string and attaching a pull string.

  B. Cardboard tunnel to crawl through   Cut ends off large cardboard boxes and attach several boxes together to make a tunnel.

C. **Climbing stairs.**

D. **Walking board**   Rest a board 1 foot wide by 3 feet long on bricks. Encourage the child to walk forward, backward, sideways, and jump down. As the child's coordination increases, decrease the width of the board.

E. **Throwing and catching a ball or bean bag**   Make a large ball out of two pieces of cloth sewn together and stuffed with rags, cotton, nylons, etc.

F. **Sand play** (using unbreakable things)

   1. Use an inner tube as the outside frame for a sandbox and fill the inside area with sand.

   2. Give the child spoons, cans, bowls, boxes, cups, sieves, and funnels to fill and dump.

   3. Cut a bleach bottle in half. Use bottom for a pail (make a handle out of heavy string); use the top for a funnel.

G. **Water play**, outdoors in a large tub or inside in the sink or bathtub. Give the child unbreakable containers, sponges, cork, bar of soap.

H. **Riding a tricycle.**

IV. **Fine motor development**

A. **Fill-'n'-dump toys**   As the child's coordination increases, decrease the size of the container and the opening (e.g., plastic milk bottle, small jars and cans) and give him smaller objects to put into the container (e.g., buttons, bottle caps, peas, beans, macaroni).

B. **Sorting activity**   Give the child three containers and bottle caps, buttons, and beans and have him put all the caps in one container, buttons in another, and beans in the other. Later use the sections of an egg carton.

C. **Stacking toys**   Build a pyramid with different-sized boxes or cans, the largest on the bottom and the smallest on top.

D. **Nesting toys**   Use graduated-sized boxes, bowls, pots, pans, cups, etc., that fit inside one another. Start by using three sizes.

E. **Clothespins and a coffee can or loaf pan**   Have the child put the clothespins on the edge of the can. This can also be used as a sorting activity; paint the pins different colors and have child sort them by color.

F. **Blocks**   Make different-sized blocks from boxes and wood scraps. Cut off the tops of two thoroughly washed milk or cream cartons and push them together. Show the child how to build. Have him copy what you build.

G. **Stringing objects**   Use old shoe laces or heavy string and spools of different sizes. As his coordination improves, give him macaroni and small beads.

H. **Puzzles**   Make your own by pasting pictures from magazines onto cardboard and cutting it into pieces. Start with simple pictures of one object and cut into three to five large pieces. With an older child, use a more complex picture and five to 10 small pieces.

I. **Large pencil or crayon**   Have the child copy a line or simple shape you make. Allow him to draw whatever he wishes. Use this time to start teaching colors. Use paper bags or cut-up cardboard boxes to draw on.

Three to 5 Years

I. **Language development**

A. **Talk to the child**, using complete thoughts and ideas. Listen to him. Encourage him to tell you what he did during the day by asking questions.

B. **Read to him** or tell him stories.

C. **Play singing games** (e.g., "Here We Go Round the Mulberry Bush," "This Is the Way We Wash Our Clothes").

D. Encourage him to **make up stories** about pictures in books and magazines ("Once upon a time ...").

E. Play with **puppets**.

II. **Personal-social development**

A. Show him how to **dress himself**.

B. Give him **small tasks** to do around the house (e.g., set table, help clear table, sweep floor, pick up toys).

C. Allow him to experiment with dressing up and **adult role playing**.

1. Let him use old clothes, cooking utensils, house-cleaning equipment, and safe tools.

2. Put chairs together to play train or bus.

3. Make a house under a table.

4. Use paper plates decorated with colored paper, ribbon, or paint to make hats.

5. Use paper bags to make hats and masks.

D. Grow plants in cans.

E. Encourage him to play **outdoor games with peers** (e.g., red rover, hide and seek).

III. Gross motor development

A. Cardboard tunnel.

B. Walking board   Use a board about 4 inches wide.

C. Sand play   Encourage child to build creatively, make cities, etc.

D. Water play   Let child enjoy washing dishes or clothes.

E. Throwing, catching, and batting a ball   Use a small rubber or semi-hard ball.

F. Throwing a bean bag at a target   Fill an old sock with beans and se_ the end shut (reinforce by sewing it several times). Make a target out of a cardboard box folded like an inverted V (tent-shaped); atta_ a heavy string to each side to stabilize it. Cut a hole in one side of the target and paint or color a clown's face around the hole.

G. Rope ladder   Make a ladder out of rope and attach it to a low bran_ of a tree for the child to climb.

H. Playing jump rope and hopscotch (start between 5 and 6 years of ag_

I. Riding a tricycle and bicycle.

IV. Fine motor development

A. Fill-'n'-dump toys.

B. Stacking toys   Increase the number and use smaller objects to be stacked (e.g., thread spools).

C. Nesting toys   Increase the number and sizes of objects to be nested_

D. Sorting activity   Give the child many objects and ask him to sort them according to color, shape, or function. For example, give the child an egg carton or small cans and colored buttons and have him sort according to color.

E. Blocks Give him blocks of different sizes and encourage him to build more complicated structures, e.g., houses, farms, forts.

F. Stringing objects String macaroni or straws cut into small pieces. Make necklaces and bracelets and paint them bright colors.

G. Puzzles Make more complicated puzzles, using detailed pictures cut into eight to 20 pieces.

H. Pencils and crayons Use paper bags or cut-up cardboard boxes to draw on. Draw a simple picture and have him color it. Draw simple forms (circles, squares, cross, etc.) and have the child copy them. Encourage the child to draw his own pictures.

I. Finger painting

1. Use the want-ad section of newspaper (because it has small, all-over print) or shelf paper for painting paper.

2. Old shirts or blouses make good smocks.

3. Recipe for paint

   1½ cups laundry starch
   1 quart boiling water
   1½ cups soap flakes
   Few drops food coloring
   ½ cup talcum powder (optional)

   Mix starch with enough cold water to make a paste, add boiling water, and stir until clear and glossy. Add talcum. Cool mixture. Add soap flakes, and stir until evenly distributed. Mixture should be thick. Add a few drops of food coloring. Pour into jar and cover. Store in a cool place.

J. Clay or Play Dough

1. Show the child how to make objects and animals.

2. Recipe for Play Dough

   1 part flour
   1 part salt
   1 part water

   Mix together to a soft consistency. Will keep 3—4 days if wrapped in wax paper and stored in the refrigerator.

K. Collages

1. Paste bits of styrofoam, cotton, cloth, colorful yarn, ribbon, paper, calendars, catalogues, magazines, pipe cleaners, etc., to a piece of cardboard to create a picture. Hang in a place for peopl to admire.

2. Paste recipe: To a handful of flour add water, a little at a time, until mixture is gooey (should be quite thick so it will not run all over the page). Add a pinch of salt.

L. Sewing cards Draw a design or picture on a piece of cardboard. Punch holes along the line. Give the child an old shoelace or large needle and yarn to sew with, along the outline.

M. Child's blunt scissors

1. Show child how to hold and use scissors.

2. Give him a long strip of paper ¾-inch wide marked with thick lines at 1-inch intervals. Have him cut off sections with one snip

3. When he is older give him wider strips sectioned off in large piec that require several strokes of the scissors.

4. Have the child practice cutting curves. When this is mastered, h can cut circles and other objects.

5. Have him cut zig-zag strips, which become crowns, mountains, Christmas trees, etc.

6. Draw large simple geometric shapes and have him cut them out.

N. Materials for construction Give him wood scraps and nails and hel him build things.

PERIODIC HEALTH SCREENING (Adult)

I. **Value of periodic health assessment** The value of periodic screening and examinations of well patients remains controversial. Few studies have shown benefit from screening procedures, or that a yearly health assessment in itself does more than introduce patients into a health ca system. Nevertheless, it has been the experience of most programs tha a periodic meeting between patient and provider is beneficial. In keep ing with this conclusion, we have developed an age-related assessment that includes the most widely recognized screening procedures plus maneuvers that are accepted because they provide baseline informatio

II. **Use of the adult health maintenance flow sheet** The guide to the
pediatric health maintenance flow sheet describes in detail the objectives
and operation of that instrument. The following is a brief but similar
outline. on the use of the adult health maintenance flow sheet (Fig. 1-2).

A. On the first visit perform the age-related tasks required for this
visit.

B. Record the date (month and year) and results, use a check if no
result is indicated.

C. Write the date of the next scheduled assessment in the top box of
the next column.

D. Outline in red the boxes of the procedures that need to be done at
the next health maintenance visit.

E. If a procedure is done before the next scheduled assessment, record
the date and result in the appropriate red-outlined box.

F. This sequence continues at each health maintenance visit. Interval
visits occurring for reasons of illness are not recorded on this sheet;
nevertheless, this sheet can be used as a reminder to accomplish certain procedures that may be omitted in acute or chronic care of
illness.

G. If an indicated procedure is not done or needs to be repeated, the
appropriate box of the next assessment is outlined in red at each
visit until the procedure is done.

Note The information recorded on the flow sheet does not supplant
the notes to be written in the body of the patient's medical chart.
However, this tabular format should simplify audit of required health
maintenance procedures.

Assessments	Date scheduled					
Females: every yr	Date seen					
Males	Age					
Age 20–45: every 5 yr	Provider					
Age 46–65: every 2 yr						
Over 65: every yr						
Complete history (once)	√					
Complete physical (once)	√					
Immunization: diphtheria-tetanus toxoid (booster every 10 yr)	Date					
1. Initial series completed	1.					
2. Last booster	2.					
Tuberculin (tine) test (once)	Date					
	Pos./Neg.					
Syphilis serology (once)	Date					
	NR/R					
Hematocrit (every assess.)	Result					
Chemical urinalysis (every assess.)	Pos./Neg.					
Blood pressure (every assess.)	Result					
Weight (every assess.)	Result					
Pap smear (every assess.)	Class					
Breast examination (every assess.)	Pos./Neg.					
Creatinine (once)	Result					
Rectal examination (every assess. after age 45); Stool guaiac	Pos./Neg.					
ECG (once after age 35)	√					
Chest x-ray (once after age 35)	√					
Health education (every assess.)						
Nutrition	√					
Physical care	√					
Behavior/psychosocial	√					
Safety	√					
Sex	√					
Tobacco/alcohol	√					
Additional tests						

Figure 1-2 Adult Health Maintenance Flow Sheet (20 Years and Over)

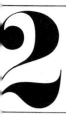

ANAPHYLAXIS (Pediatric and Adult)

I. **Definition** A hypersensitivity reaction usually occurring within seconds to minutes after exposure to an antigen. The reaction ranges from mild self-limited symptoms to rapid death.

II. **Etiology** Agents commonly associated with anaphylaxis include the following. This list is not exhaustive.

   A. **Antibiotics** (especially penicillin and its semisynthetic derivatives).

   B. **Biologicals**

   1. Nonhuman serums.

   2. Gamma globulin.

   3. Influenza vaccine.

   4. Tetanus toxoid.

   5. Measles and other egg-based vaccines.

   C. **Injectable medications**

   1. Imferon (iron dextran injection).

   2. Dextran.

   D. **Local anesthetics.**

   E. **Aspirin.**

   F. **Hymenoptera stings** (bee, yellow jacket, wasp, and hornet).

   G. **Allergic extracts** (skin-testing and treatment solutions).

   H. **Foods** (especially eggs, nuts, and shellfish).

   I. **Intravenous narcotics** (heroin).

   Note Generally, agents administered parenterally are more likely to result in life-threatening or fatal anaphylactic reactions than those ingested orally or administered topically to mucous membranes. Medications administered orally, such as aspirin or penicillin, however, have been associated with fatal reactions.

III. **Clinical features**   Anaphylaxis is usually characterized by some or all of the following sequence of signs and symptoms. The sooner symptoms develop after the initiating stimulus, the more intense the reaction.

   A. Generalized flush.

   B. Urticaria.

   C. Paroxysmal coughing.

   D. Severe anxiety.

   E. Dyspnea.

   F. Wheezing.

   G. Orthopnea.

   H. Vomiting.

   I. Cyanosis.

   J. Shock.

IV. **Laboratory studies**   None.

V. **Differential diagnosis**   The development of symptoms and signs within minutes after contact with an antigen, especially a parenterally administered antigen, makes the diagnosis of anaphylaxis almost certain. An anxiety reaction to an injection might produce some of the symptoms, but consideration of that diagnosis should not result in more than momentary delay in instituting treatment for anaphylaxis.

VI. **Treatment**

   A. **Prevention**

   1. Before administering or prescribing any medication, inquire carefully for a history of reactions. **Note**   Anaphylactoid reactions can occur without prior sensitization.

   2. Minimize the use of biologic products (e.g., horse antiserum, unnecessary boosters of tetanus toxoid).

   3. After receiving an agent capable of inducing anaphylaxis (e.g., injection of penicillin, allergy vaccine) the patient should be required to remain in the clinic for at least 15 minutes.

   4. If a patient is allergic to insect venom, he should be counseled to wear a medical alert bracelet, not to go barefoot, to avoid fields of flowers, ripe fruit, bright-colored clothing and perfume during

warm weather, and to carry a kit containing epinephrine and a syringe for injection.

B. **Immediate treatment** Symptoms beginning within 15 minutes after administration of the inciting agent require the most expedient management.

1. **Tourniquet** If an injection has been given into an extremity, a tourniquet should immediately be applied proximal to the site to obstruct venous return from the injection.

2. **Aqueous epinephrine 1:1000**

   a. **Pediatric dose** 0.01 ml per kg (0.005 ml per lb), maximum single dose 0.3 ml.

   b. **Adult dose** 0.3−0.5 ml.

   c. Inject dose (**a** or **b**) subcutaneously into the upper arm and massage area. Repeat same dose in 5 minutes if necessary.

   d. Also inject the same dose (**a** or **b**) one time below the tourniquet around the site of the offending injection or sting to decrease absorption of antigen.

   Note If the patient is in shock give aqueous epinephrine 1:10,000 (1 ml of 1:1000 diluted with 9 ml of IV fluid) intravenously.

   a. **Pediatric dose** 1:10,000 aqueous epinephrine: 0.1 ml per kg (0.05 ml per lb), maximum dose 3 ml.

   b. **Adult dose** 1:10,000 aqueous epinephrine: 3−5 ml.

3. **Airway** Maintain airway and administer oxygen by mask. Hypoxia can result from hypotension and upper airway edema.

4. **Intravenous therapy** Start an intravenous infusion and be prepared to administer the following supportive therapy if patient fails to respond to initial therapy or is in shock when first seen. *Steps 1−3 should always be done first.*

   a. **Shock** Give intravenous fluid (normal saline solution, lactated Ringer's solution, or plasma volume expander) *rapidly* to support blood pressure. In anaphylaxis, shock results from vasodilation and subsequent inadequate plasma volume.

      (1) **Pediatric dose** 20 ml per kg (10 ml per lb) over 15−30 minutes, then slow to 10 ml per kg (5 ml per lb) per hour.

        (2) **Adult dose** 1000 ml per 15–30 minutes.

    b. **Bronchospasm** Give aminophylline solution intravenously *after shock is controlled.*

        (1) **Pediatric dose** 6 mg per kg (3 mg per lb) diluted in two equal volumes of IV fluid and administered over 10 minutes.

        (2) **Adult dose** 500 mg in 20 ml of IV fluid over 10 minutes

5. **Record** Maintain a flow sheet with time, vital signs, and medications administered.

6. **Consultation** Contact physician for further therapeutic guidance but do not allow the patient to be left alone.

VII. Complications

A. **Upper airway obstruction** Pharyngeal, uvular, or laryngeal edema, or any combination of these, can develop acutely, especially in children. Observe pharynx frequently. Be prepared to insert oral or endotracheal airway.

B. **Lower airway obstruction** Bronchospasm in children may be so severe that decreased tidal volume makes wheezing inaudible.

C. **Hypotension** Frequent pulse and blood pressure determinations should be done.

D. **Cardiac arrhythmias** Arrhythmias may arise owing to hypoxia, especially in adults.

E. **Aspiration of gastric contents** In children, vomiting often accompanies anaphylaxis.

F. **Hypoxic seizures.**

G. **Cardiac arrest.**

VIII. Consultation – referral
After instituting immediate therapy (**VI.B**), contact physician for further therapy and disposition.

IX. Follow-up

A. An allergy label should be placed on the front cover of the patient's medical record.

B. If the reaction was to an insect sting, the patient should be referred for desensitization. Follow up should be done to ensure that desensitization is instituted and that preventive measures (see **VI.A.4**) are being taken.

ANIMAL BITES (Pediatric and Adult)

I. **Definition and etiology**   Bites of any animal, provoked or unprovoked, excluding snakes (see Snake Bites [Pediatric and Adult]).

II. **Clinical features**

A. **Symptoms**   Few other than pain at site of bite.

B. **Signs**   Puncture wounds or lacerations.

III. **Laboratory studies**   Culture of infected bites.

IV. **Differential diagnosis**   The chief concern is the possibility of rabies in the offending animal.   Unprovoked bites must be treated with more suspicion than bites from teased or taunted animals.

A. Any mammal may carry rabies.

B. The dog is no longer the chief carrier in the United States.   In certain localities other animals, such as skunks, foxes, raccoons, bats, and cows, are at least as likely to carry rabies as dogs are.

C. The virus is contained in the saliva of the infected animal and transmitted to the wound by the teeth penetrating the skin; thus, scratch and abrasion do not transmit virus.

D. Rabbits, squirrels, chipmunks, rats, and mice are seldom infective.

E. Properly vaccinated animals have only a slight chance of developing the disease.

V. **Treatment**

A. Immediately wash the wound with copious amounts of soap and water.   Then carefully wash away all traces of soap and wash with Zephiran (benzalkonium chloride) solution.   (Zephiran is inactivated by soap.)   Alcohol, 40–70%, may be substituted for Zephiran.

B. Control bleeding.

C. Carry out tetanus prophylaxis in clean wounds.

1. If no previous immunization, begin series of primary immunization.

2. If incomplete immunization, complete series of primary immunization.

3. If no booster in 5 years, give 0.5 ml tetanus toxoid IM.

D. Rabies prophylaxis; consult physician.   Therapy only after consultation.   There appear to be benefits from beginning immunization as soon as possible if a risk of rabies is present.

VI. Complications

   A. Infection at wound site.

   B. Rarely, tetanus.

   C. Rabies.

VII. Consultation – referral

   A. All bites in which there is reasonable suspicion of rabies.

   B. All large or dirty bites for instructions, wound management, and rabies and tetanus prophylaxis.

VIII. Follow-up   As recommended by consultant.

SNAKE BITES (Pediatric and Adult)

   I. **Definition**   Snake bites can be classified as those caused by:

   A. Nonpoisonous snakes.

   B. Poisonous snakes but with no venenation (injection of venom).

   C. Poisonous snakes with venenation.

   II. **Etiology** (snakes native to the United States)

   A. **Pit vipers**

   1. **Varieties**

      a. **Rattlesnake**   Eastern and western diamondbacks are most frequently associated with human bites and are found throughout the United States.

      b. **Copperhead moccasin**   This is found in southern United States usually in the highland.

      c. **Water, or cottonmouth, moccasin**   This is found in southern swamps.

   2. **Description**

      a. All have **triangular-shaped heads**.

      b. All have a **pit** between each eye and nostril.

      c. All have **elliptical** (rather than round) **pupils**.

      d. **Other features**   Rattlesnakes have rattles on the end of their tails. Water moccasins have a white mouth.

3. **Severity**   Rattlesnake bites generally are more serious than those of other species, mainly because of the amount of venom injected by its bite.

B. **Eastern coral snake**

1. **Location**   Florida, coastal Georgia, and the coastal Carolinas.

2. **Description**   This is a small red and black striped snake with yellow rings separating red from black. Its nose is black, and it does not have a noticeable neck or a spade- or triangular-shaped head. It may be confused with the nonpoisonous garter snake, which does not have a black nose.

3. **Severity**   Venom is very toxic and affects the nervous system. Fortunately, the snake is shy and rarely bites.

III. **Clinical features of pit viper bites** (Eastern coral snakes cause almost no local symptoms, and systemic symptoms are slow to develop.)

A. **Symptoms** (with venenation)

1. Pain at site of bite.

2. Paresthesias of affected part.

3. General weakness.

4. Faintness and dizziness.

5. Nausea, vomiting, and diarrhea.

B. **Signs**

1. **General** (if severe venenation)

a. Hypotension.

b. Sweating.

2. **Local**

a. Puncture wound.

b. Swelling and edema.

c. Erythema.

d. Ecchymoses.

C. **Gradation of wounds**

1. **Grade 0 (no venenation)**   Minimal pain and less than 1 inch of surrounding edema and erythema. No systemic involvement.

2. **Grade 1 (minimal venenation)**   Severe pain, and 1–5 inches of surrounding edema and erythema in the first 12 hours after the bite. *No* systemic involvement.

3. **Grade 2 (moderate venenation)**   Severe pain and edema, petechi and ecchymosis of entire extremity. Sometimes, systemic involv ment, e.g., nausea, vomiting, giddiness, shock, and neurotoxic symptoms (ptosis, weakness, abnormal reflexes).

4. **Grade 3 (severe venenation)**   Severe pain, edema of entire extremity, and generalized petechiae and ecchymoses. Systemic symptoms appear rapidly.

IV. **Laboratory studies**   None are necessary before consultation with physician.

V. **Differential diagnosis**

A. **Poisonous versus nonpoisonous snake.**

B. **Venenation versus nonvenenation** (Pit vipers may not venenate, particularly if the snake has just eaten or struck another object.) If the wound is more than 1 hour old and there is no local edema, pain, or tenderness, then venenation has not occurred.

VI. **Treatment**

A. **All snake bites** (including those of nonpoisonous snakes)

1. Clean wound with antiseptic solution (e.g., Zephiran [benzalko-nium chloride], Betadine [povidone-iodine]) or with soap and water.

2. Carry out tetanus prophylaxis, depending on immunization statu (see Animal Bites [Pediatric and Adult], **V.C**).

B. **Pit viper bites**

1. **Bites seen within 1 hour**   Administer first aid for all grades of bites seen within 1 hour and suspected of being made by a poison ous snake.

a. Apply a tourniquet above the site of the bite.

b. Make a single longitudinal incision 1/8–1/4 inch in length through the fang marks and about 1/4-inch deep or as deep as the fang mark. Apply mechanical suction over the incision for at least 15 minutes.

2. **Bites seen after 1 hour**   (Steps **1a** and **b** are no longer helpful and should not be done.)

a. Keep patient quiet and lying down.

b. Do *not* pack extremity in ice or ice water.

c. Do *not* give patient alcohol.

d. Monitor blood pressure, pulse, and respiratory rate every one-half hour.

e. Be prepared to treat shock.

3. **Specific therapy**   Consult physician first, if possible.

   a. **Grade 0**   No antivenin.

   b. **Grade 1**   1 ampule (10 ml) polyvalent crotaline antivenin (Wyeth) IV slow push. Do sensitivity test first (see **e**).

   c. **Grade 2**   3–4 ampules (30–40 ml) antivenin IV slow push. Do sensitivity test first (see **e**).

   d. **Grade 3**   5 ampules (50 ml) antivenin IV slow push. Do sensitivity test first (see **e**).

   e. **Sensitivity test**

      (1)   Antivenin is a horse serum and can cause immediate anaphylaxis and a delayed serum sickness reaction. Sensitivity testing is done to see if a person is susceptible to anaphylaxis.

      (2)   Dilute the antivenin to 1:100 (1 drop of serum in 5 ml of sterile saline or water) and put one drop of this mixture onto the conjunctiva of one eye. Put one drop of saline in the other eye as a control. If there is no reaction (injection of vessels, itching, edema of the eyelid), give antivenin IV. If there is a reaction, consult physician before giving any antivenin.

C. **Coral snake bites**

   1. Any person bitten by a coral snake who has a break in the skin from teeth or fangs should be referred to a physician and observed for 48 hours.

   2. If there are fang marks, wash the lesion and apply a tourniquet until consultation can be obtained.

   3. Refer to a physician and obtain North American coral snake antivenin (Wyeth Laboratories).

VII. **Complications**

    A. Respiratory depression.

    B. Cardiovascular collapse.

    C. Coma.

    D. Local necrosis.

    E. Infection of wound.

    F. Joint disability.

    G. Loss of digits or extremity.

VIII. **Consultation – referral**   All snake bites.

IX. **Follow-up**   All persons receiving antivenin should be told of the possible symptoms of serum sickness (malaise, arthralgia, urticaria, swellin of lymph nodes, fever). Should any of these develop after the patient discharged from the clinic (usually within 8–12 days), he should retur

MINOR BURNS (Pediatric and Adult)

I. **Definition**   Thermal injuries to the skin, which may be

    A. **First degree**   Erythema only.

    B. **Second degree (partial thickness)**   Blister formation with or withou peeling and weeping.

    C. **Third degree (full thickness)**   Early, may have charred or whitish appearance and areas of anesthesia.

II. **Etiology**   Contact with any heat source. The degree of damage depen on the duration of exposure and the source of heat. Scalds generally cause second-degree burns, whereas flame or hot metal may cause thir degree burns.

III. **Clinical features**

    A. **Symptoms**   Usually only pain. Severe burns with nerve damage ma be less painful than first- or second-degree burns.

    B. **Signs**   See I.

IV. **Laboratory studies**   None.

V. **Differential diagnosis**   In pediatric age group consider child abuse or neglect.

VI. Treatment

A. First degree   No treatment necessary.

B. Second degree

1. Clean gently with soap and water.

2. Leave blisters intact.

3. Cover burned area with Furacin gauze and bulky dry sterile dressing.

4. Carry out tetanus prophylaxis:

   a. If no previous immunization, begin series of primary immunization.

   b. If incomplete immunization, complete series of primary immunization.

   c. If no booster in 5 years, give 0.5 ml tetanus toxoid IM.

C. Third degree   Refer to physician in all cases.

VII. Complications

A. Bacterial infection.

B. Progression of second to third degree, if infection develops.

VIII. Consultation — referral

A. All third-degree burns totally or partially involving the burned area.

B. Extensive second-degree burns, involving an area greater than that covered by examiner's hand.

C. Facial burns.

D. Any suspicion of child abuse or neglect.

IX. Follow-up

A. First degree   None.

B. Second degree

1. Have the patient return in 2 days for dressing change.

2. Have the patient return every 1–2 days thereafter until epithelialization occurs without infection.

CARDIAC ARREST (Adult)

I. **Definition**   The cessation of effective cardiac function due to either a failure of electrical excitation (cardiac standstill) or an arrhythmia that does not permit effective ventricular contraction (e.g., ventricular fibrillation).

II. **Etiology**   Cardiac arrest may be associated with any severe illness but in an ambulatory setting it usually occurs in persons with acute or chronic cardiac or respiratory disease, for example:

   A. Arteriosclerotic heart disease with or without myocardial infarction

   B. Chronic obstructive pulmonary disease.

III. **Clinical features**

   A. **Symptoms**   Associated with underlying disease.

   B. **Signs**

   1. Poor or absent blood pressure and pulses.

   2. Unconsciousness.

   3. Absent or gasping respirations.

   4. Cyanosis.

IV. **Laboratory studies**   During the acute episode surrounding a cardiac arrest there is no need for laboratory determinations.

V. **Differential diagnosis**   See II.

VI. **Treatment**   Ultimately treatment depends on the etiology; however, initially there are certain things that must be done once one has determined that there is no blood pressure and heartbeat is either absent or irregular and ineffective.   If a physician is not present and the patient is a candidate for resuscitation, the nurse should begin the following measures with assistance from other clinic personnel.

   A. **Pulmonary treatment**   Examine the airway for foreign objects, insert a mouthpiece that holds the tongue forward (make sure the tongue not obstructing the airway), and begin assisted respiration with an Ambu bag.   Attach oxygen to the bag as soon as possible.   If no Ambu bag is available, mouth-to-mouth resuscitation must be used and is sufficient temporarily.   Suction is helpful if secretions are present in the mouth and throat.

   Note   These two steps together will frequently reestablish a heartbeat.

B. **Cardiac massage (external)**   Begin cardiac massage in a ratio of 5 heartbeats per breath.* The hands should be placed on the sternum so that downward pressure will compress the heart between the sternum and the spinal column. Each beat should be deliberate at a rate of approximately 1 per second and done with relatively stiff arms, pressure being applied through the heels of the hands from the shoulders. As massage is difficult to perform against a soft mattress, a board should be placed under the patient's back. If a board is unavailable, the patient should be transferred to the floor. Evaluate the success of cardiac massage by palpating a large artery, such as the femoral artery. External cardiac massage should generate a pulse.

C. **Defibrillation**   If (1) no pulse or heartbeat is detectable, (2) an airway has been established and oxygen therapy begun, (3) a blow to the sternum has not generated a heartbeat, and (4) the situation is such that ventricular fibrillation is likely, defibrillation may be tried, if a defibrillator is readily available and someone trained in its use is present.

   1. Continue external cardiac massage and assisted respiration until defibrillation.

   2. When bedside is clear, defibrillate at 400 watt-seconds.

D. **Treatment without defibrillation**   If there is no defibrillator available or no one present trained in its use, maintain external cardiac massage and assisted respiration.

   1. Place an intravenous line:

      a. Start

         (1)   Normal saline solution

               or

         (2)   5% dextrose in water

               or

         (3)   Any available standard IV solution. The main purpose of using fluids is to keep the IV tube open and available for medicines.

      b. As acidosis occurs in tissues without adequate perfusion, give sodium bicarbonate, 89.2 mEq (2 ampules), IV. Repeat at 5—10 minute intervals as long as resuscitation continues.

*See supplement to *J.A.M.A.,* Vol. 227, No. 1, Feb. 18, 1974.

2. Begin electrocardiography and the following treatment:

a. No heartbeat (asystole)

(1) Blow to the chest.

(2) 1:800 epinephrine, 5 ml intracardiac.

b. Complexes without a pulse

(1) 10% calcium chloride, 10 ml IV.

(2) Isoproterenol (Isuprel), drip IV at 10 μg per minute.

c. Ventricular fibrillation (in this situation chemical intervention is of little use)

(1) Lidocaine, 50 mg IV in a bolus.

(2) If **(1)** does not stop fibrillation, repeat or increase to 100 mg IV in a bolus.

E. **Final steps**   Resuscitation may continue until heartbeat and adequate respirations begin. The patient then should be transferred to a hospital, as soon as a vehicle with support equipment is available.

VII. Complications

A. Death.

B. Central nervous system damage from hypoxia.

C. Renal tubular necrosis.

VIII. Consultation — referral   All patients after lifesaving measures have been initiated.

IX. Follow-up   Varies with each patient.

CONVULSIONS (Pediatric)

I. **Definition**   Tonic or clonic muscular contractions, or both, usually associated with unconsciousness. They are expressions of abnormal electrical discharge of neurons in the central nervous system (CNS).

A. The terms *convulsions, seizures, epilepsy,* and *fits* may be used synonymously by patients.

B. This definition applies to major motor convulsions only. Any unexplained, episodic alteration of consciousness could represent a seizure or abnormal electrical discharge in the CNS.

II. **Etiology** (incomplete list)

   A. **Neonatal period**

      1. Anoxic CNS injury.

      2. Birth trauma.

      3. CNS infection.

      4. Hypoglycemia.

      5. Hypocalcemia.

      6. Congenital abnormalities of the CNS.

   B. **Infancy**

      1. Febrile convulsions.

      2. CNS infection.

      3. Residual damage from neonatal causes.

      4. CNS trauma.

      5. Ingestion of drugs and poisons.

      6. Breath-holding spell causing anoxia.

   C. **Childhood**

      1. Idiopathic epilepsy.

      2. Residual damage from neonatal causes.

      3. CNS infection.

      4. Ingestion of drugs and poisons.

      5. CNS trauma.

      6. Glomerulonephritis.

III. **Clinical features** (depend to some extent on age and etiology)

   A. **Symptoms**

      1. Sometimes, short prodrome of irritability, anorexia, headache, and lethargy.

      2. Symptoms characterizing underlying disorder.

   B. **Signs** (usual sequential evolution; may be great variation, however, depending in part on underlying disorder)

1. Usually, abrupt onset of tonic muscular contraction.

2. Tonic spasm often occurring simultaneously with loss of consciousness.

3. Facial pallor, often followed by erythema and then cyanosis, depending on length of tonic spasm of respiratory muscles.

4. Eyeballs rolled upward or to one side.

5. Head hyperextended or turned to one side. Contraction of facial muscles leading to contorted expression.

6. Abdominal and chest muscles in tonic spasm, often accompanied by urination and occasionally by defecation.

7. Clonic phase (rhythmic contraction of muscles), localized or generalized and lasting for a variable period of time.

8. Often, sleep or lethargy.

IV. **Laboratory studies** After consultation. Tests depend on suspected underlying cause. (Save blood for glucose determination before giving glucose.)

V. **Differential diagnosis**

A. Tremulousness associated with high fever or chill, or both.

B. Hysterical episodes. Hypoglycemia can cause behavior disturbances as well as convulsions, however.

C. Breath-holding spell causing unconsciousness. Occasionally breath-holding spell can lead to enough anoxia to cause a convulsion.

VI. **Treatment** In the great majority of cases convulsions are self-limited and cease before treatment is instituted. Occasionally more harm is done by overtreatment than by observation.

A. **General measures**

1. Maintain a clear airway by turning the patient on one side with head low to encourage gravity drainage of secretions and vomitus and to prevent aspiration. Suction when necessary.

2. Give oxygen for cyanosis.

3. Place the patient in such a position as to prevent injury by falling or knocking against objects.

4. Do *not* try to pry clenched jaws apart to place an object between

5. Observe and be able to describe the duration and focal elements of the convulsion. Focal elements include:

   a. Unusual behavior before the convulsion.

   b. Movements of one part or side of the body early or late in the convulsion.

   c. Persistent weakness of one part of the body after the convulsion has occurred.

B. Specific therapy

1. **History**   Obtain a brief history sufficient to discover any etiologic disorder that will respond to specific therapy, for example:

   a. Insulin-induced hypoglycemia.

   b. Intracranial hemorrhage caused by head trauma.

   c. Hyponatremia from treatment of prolonged diarrhea by non-sodium-containing fluids.

   d. High fever prior to convulsion.

   e. Renal disease suggesting hypertensive encephalopathy.

2. **Anticonvulsants**

   a. **Paraldehyde** should be administered *rectally* under the following circumstances:

      (1)   A convulsion has lasted for more than 10 minutes

      or

      (2)   Three or more separate convulsions have occurred in the preceding 30 minutes.

      Mix the dose of paraldehyde (see Table 2-1) with an equal volume of mineral oil and give as a retention enema.

   b. **Phenobarbital** should be administered intramuscularly (see Table 2-2) under the following circumstances:

      (1)   A convulsion has not stopped within 30 minutes after rectal administration of paraldehyde

      or

      (2)   A second convulsion starts within 30 minutes after rectal administration of paraldehyde

Table 2-1 Rectal Dose of Paraldehyde per Body Weight, as an Anticonvulsa

Body Weight	Paraldehyde (ml)
3–5 kg (6–10 lb)	1.2
5–7 kg (10–15 lb)	1.8
7–9 kg (15–20 lb)	2.4
9–11 kg (20–24 lb)	3.0
11–13 kg (24–29 lb)	3.6
13–15 kg (29–33 lb)	4.2
15–17 kg (33–37 lb)	4.8
17–19 kg (37–42 lb)	5.4
Over 19 kg (over 42 lb)	6.0

and

(3) A physician consultation is still not available.

3. **Transfer of patient** If a physician consultation is still not available at the time the phenobarbital is given, consideration should be given to transfer of the patient, accompanied by trained personnel, to a facility where a physician is available.

VII. **Complications**

A. Aspiration of vomitus causing pneumonitis or lung abscess.

B. Prolonged anoxia causing CNS injury.

C. Traumatic injury during convulsion.

D. Complications of the underlying disorder.

VIII. **Consultation – referral** A physician should be consulted concerning a patients with convulsions, even if they stop spontaneously before arriv in the clinic. Therapy may be started while the consultant is being contacted.

IX. **Follow-up** As recommended by consultant.

CONVULSIONS (Adult)

I. **Definition** Clonic or tonic muscular contractions, or both, usually ass ciated with unconsciousness. Contractions are often accompanied by salivation and incontinence.

II. Etiology

A. Epilepsy

1. Initial onset may occur in adulthood but most frequently happens in childhood and puberty.

2. Seizure in a known epileptic.

B. Drug withdrawal (most commonly barbiturates).

C. Alcohol withdrawal   Usually short-lived and occurring as one seizure or repeated seizures within a space of a few hours.

D. Hypoglycemia   The effects of hypoglycemia on CNS range from inappropriate behavior to confusion to coma.

E. Hypertensive encephalopathy.

F. Cardiac arrhythmia   Seizures associated with arrhythmias are usually short-lived and generally have only the tonic component.

G. Expanding brain lesion.

II. Clinical features

A. Symptoms

1. History of:

Table 2-2 Intramuscular Dose of Phenobarbital per Body Weight, as an Anticonvulsant

Weight	Phenobarbital (mg)	Volume (ml) of a 130 mg per ml Solution
3−4 kg (7−9 lb)	20	0.15
4−5 kg (9−11 lb)	25	0.19
5−6 kg (11−13 lb)	30	0.23
6−7 kg (13−15 lb)	35	0.27
7−9 kg (15−20 lb)	45	0.34
9−11 kg (20−24 lb)	55	0.42
11−13 kg (24−29 lb)	65	0.50
13−16 kg (29−35 lb)	80	0.62
16−19 kg (35−42 lb)	95	0.73
19−22 kg (42−49 lb)	110	0.85
22−26 kg (49−57 lb)	130	1.00
26−31 kg (57−68 lb)	155	1.20
31−37 kg (68−82 lb)	185	1.40
Over 37 kg (over 82 lb)	195	1.50

      a. Epilepsy.

      b. Use of insulin or oral hypoglycemic agents.

      c. Hypertension.

      d. Alcohol or drug abuse.

      e. Situational problems and emotional stress, particularly in young females.

    2. No obvious cause.

    3. Classic cry at beginning of epilepsy seizure.

B. Signs (usual sequential evolution: may have great variation, however, depending in part on underlying disorder)

    1. Usually abrupt onset of tonic muscular contraction.

    2. Tonic spasm often occurring simultaneously with loss of consciousness.

    3. Facial pallor, often followed by erythema and then cyanosis, depending on length of tonic spasm of respiratory muscles.

    4. Eyeballs rolled upward or to one side.

    5. Head hyperextended or turned to one side. Contraction of facial muscles leading to contorted expression.

    6. Abdominal and chest muscles in tonic spasm, often accompanied by urination and occasionally by defecation.

    7. Clonic phase (rhythmic contraction of muscles), localized or generalized and lasting for a variable period of time.

    8. Often, sleep or lethargy.

IV. Laboratory studies None necessary in the case of an actively convulsing patient.

V. Differential diagnosis

  A. See **II.**

  B. Occasionally a hysterical patient may mimic movements of a convulsion.

VI. Treatment

  A. History of a seizure Refer to physician for:

    1. Diagnosis

or

2. Regulation of drugs if seizure was in a known epileptic.

B. **Active convulsion**   Nurse practitioners should not attempt to treat convulsions alone, unless there is no alternative. The following are guidelines for treating adults until transfer or consultation is obtained. Most seizures are self-limited and may stop during evaluation. Occasionally more harm is done by overtreatment than by observation.

1. **General measures**

   a. Maintain a clear airway by turning the patient on one side with head low to encourage gravity drainage of secretions and vomitus and prevent aspiration. Suction when necessary.

   b. Give oxygen for cyanosis.

   c. Place patient in such a position as to prevent injury by falling or knocking against objects.

   d. Do *not* try to pry clenched jaws apart to place an object between the teeth.

   e. Observe and be able to describe duration and focal elements of the convulsion (see Convulsions [Pediatric] , **VI.A.5**).

   f. Monitor respirations, blood pressure, temperature, and pulse.

2. **Specific therapy**   If after assessment patient is still having seizure:

   a. Start IV infusion.

   b. Give 20 ml of 50% glucose IV.

   If no response in 5 minutes:

   c. Give 10 mg of diazepam (Valium) IV.

   Note   *Diphenylhydantoin* takes sufficiently long for effective therapeutic action that it is not used initially to terminate seizures. One may give 0.1 gm of diphenylhydantoin IV during a seizure or orally immediately following a seizure. This is done as an adjunct to more rapidly acting anticonvulsants and to initiate maintenance therapy.

VII. **Complications**

A. Status epilepticus.

B. Aspiration.

      C. Traumatic injury during convulsion.

      D. Complications of underlying disorder.

VIII. Consultation – referral   Consult on all seizures, but therapy may be started.

  IX. Follow-up   Individualize for patient or cause of seizure.

MINOR HEAD INJURIES (Pediatric and Adult)

  I. Definition   Trauma to the head that does *not* result in any alteration cerebral function.

 II. Etiology   A blow to the head occurring in any of a host of circumstan in which either an object strikes the skull or the skull strikes an object

III. Clinical features   The nurse practitioner should manage *only* those patients having minor head injuries as defined by the following positiv and negative symptoms and signs.

  A. Symptoms

     1. *No* loss of consciousness at time of injury.

     2. *No* alteration in sensorium from the time of injury until the pati is seen and evaluated.

     3. *No* nausea or vomiting.

     4. *No* focal neurologic symptoms.

     5. Sometimes, minimally to moderately severe headache.

  B. Signs

     1. Normal vital signs.

     2. *No* palpable defect on examination of the skull.

     3. Sometimes, localized area of tenderness over the skull.

     4. *No* discharge from the ears.

     5. *No* discharge from the nose.

     6. *No* evidence of blood.

     7. Full consciousness, alertness, and orientation to time, person, and place.

     8. Intact cranial nerves.

      9. *No* weakness on motor testing.

      10. *No* demonstrable sensory loss.

      11. Intact and symmetric reflexes.

      12. Flexor plantar response.

IV. Laboratory and other studies None indicated in minor head injury.

V. Differential diagnosis Minor head injury (see **III**) must be differentiated from all other head injuries.

VI. Treatment Careful observation. The patient *may* be allowed to go home if:

    A. There is a competent person who will assume responsibility for observing the patient carefully.

    B. Detailed written instructions as to the nature of the observations to be made are provided. Figure 2-1 is an example of the type of written instructions to be given the patient's family.

VII. Complications Even a very minor head injury such as just described can result in the severe complications of subdural or epidural hematoma and other complications, resulting in rapid deterioration of the patient's neurologic status and severe disability or death.

VIII. Consultation – referral All head injuries that do not fit the definition of a minor head injury according to these guidelines.

IX. Follow-up See **VI** and Figure 2-1.

INGESTIONS AND POISONINGS (Pediatric)

I. Definition

    A. Ingestion or absorption of any nonfoodstuff.

    B. Accidental ingestion of a medicine.

II. Etiology Almost every substance has probably been ingested by children. Commonly ingested toxic substances include aspirin, iron tablets, and petroleum products.

III. Clinical features Ingestions are most common under 5 years of age.

    A. History

      1. The ingestion is often witnessed or an empty container is found where the child could have ingested its contents.

Observation after Head Injury

The patient should be checked every 2 hours for the first 24 hours after the injury. If he is asleep, he should be awakened. If any of the following signs are noted, please call the family nurse practitioner (FNP) immediately or return the patient to the clinic as soon as possible:

1. Patient unusually sleepy or hard to wake up.
2. Patient mentally confused. Does not know who he is or where he is. Does not recognize familiar people or places.
3. Patient very restless, disturbed, or agitated. Being upset is normal after an accident, but when a patient becomes very nervous and excited after having been quiet and calm, it is important to report it.
4. Nausea and vomiting (complains of being "sick to my stomach" or of throwing up).
5. Severe headache.
6. Difference in the size of the pupils of the eyes. The pupil is the round, darkest part of the center of the eye. Normal pupils are both the same size.
7. Weakness of the arms or legs. This sign is especially important if it is only on one side of the body.
8. Fits, seizures, or convulsions.
9. Drainage of fluid from the ears or nose.

Guidelines for Care at Home

1. The patient may move around and be up as much as he desires.
2. He may eat or drink anything, except *no* alcoholic beverages.
3. If the patient takes medicines regularly, he should ask about taking these medicines after head injury.
4. For mild headache, the patient should lie flat until the headache goes away.

_____

FNP or MD

I understand the above instructions:

_____

Signed

_____

Relationship to patient

_____

Date

Figure 2-1 Instructions for home observation of a patient after head injury.

2. Ingestions are more likely to occur during periods of disruption or stress in the household.

3. Someone in the household may be on drug therapy.

4. Accidental ingestion has occurred in the past.

5. Child under 1 year of age may be receiving an excessive dose of medication.

6. Ingestion in a school-age child may be a suicide attempt if he is depressed.

B. Symptoms and signs

1. Symptoms and signs are likely to be absent if the ingestion is discovered or suspected soon after it occurred. Many ingested substances have low toxicity and will produce no symptoms or signs.

2. Poisonings and overdosage of medicines can cause a great variety of symptoms and signs, often simulating natural diseases. Consider poisoning especially under the following circumstances:

   a. Presence of historical factors (see A).

   b. Patient aged 1–4 years.

   c. Very sudden onset of symptoms.

   d. Abnormal odor to breath or clothes.

   e. Unexplained findings, especially unconsciousness, in any patient.

IV. Laboratory studies As suggested by consultant. Save vomitus, gastric contents, and urine.

V. Differential diagnosis

A. Nonaccidental ingestion

1. Suicide attempt in child over 5 years of age.

2. Child abuse or neglect.

B. Natural diseases (depending on symptoms and signs).

VI. Treatment

A. Prevention

1. Label all containers as to contents.

2. Keep medicines in safety cap containers. Always replace cap after use.

3. Lock all medicines and poisons away and out of reach of childre

4. Do not store nondrinkable or nonedible substances in drink or food containers.

5. Keep syrup of ipecac in the house.

6. Caution parents about the risks of ingestions during disruptive periods in the household, e.g., moving, house painting, emotionally stressful situations.

B. **Telephone calls about ingestion**

1. Try to determine what and how much was ingested and when it was ingested.

2. Ask that the remainder of the ingested substance and its contair be brought with the patient to the clinic. If uncertain what mig have been ingested, have all potentially ingested materials that a available in the household brought with the patient, e.g., medications.

3. *If no contraindications to vomiting exist* (see **E.2**), vomiting ma be induced before leaving home or on the way to the clinic to decrease potential toxicity. Syrup of ipecac should be available in every household as part of health maintenance procedures an may be given by parents to induce vomiting (see **E.1** for dosage)

C. **General supportive therapy** (as needed)

1. **Maintenance of airway**

   a. Suction of secretions.

   b. Head turned to side and lower than feet to avoid aspiration c vomitus.

   c. Oropharyngeal airway.

2. **Cardiopulmonary resuscitation.**

3. **Control of convulsions** (see Convulsions [Pediatric], **VI**).

4. **Treatment of shock** Start administering intravenous fluids (normal saline solution, Ringer's solution, or plasma volume expander) in a dose of 20 ml per kilogram of body weight (10 m per pound) over 15–30 minutes.

D. **Consultation** Seek consultation before further therapy if consulta is immediately available.

E. **Induction of emesis**   If consultant is not immediately available and ingestion is suspected, induce emesis with syrup of ipecac. (Do not wait for symptoms to develop.)

   1. **Dose of syrup of ipecac** to induce emesis if no contraindications are present (see **E.2**)

      a. **6 months to 1 year of age**   10 ml (2 teaspoons) followed by at least 4–6 oz of clear liquid.

      b. **Over 1 year of age**   15 ml (1 tablespoon) followed by at least 6–8 oz of clear liquid.

      Note   If child does not vomit after 20 minutes, the same dose may be repeated.

   2. **Contraindications**

      a. **Unconsciousness.**

      b. **Convulsions.**

      c. **Ingestion of corrosives** (strong alkali or acid), e.g., toilet bowl cleaners and drain cleaners, such as lye, Drano, Liquid Plumr, Saniflush. This can be suspected if burns are present on the lips or tongue or in the mouth, or there is pain on swallowing.

      d. **Ingestion of petroleum products**, e.g., kerosene, gasoline, furniture polish, cleaning fluid, paint thinner. This may be suspected by odor on the breath or clothes or by odor of the container.

VII. **Complications**   These vary depending on the substance and amount to which the patient was exposed.

VIII. **Consultation – referral**   All patients with established or suspected ingestion or poisoning.

IX. **Follow-up**   As suggested by consultant.

OVERDOSE OF SEDATIVE, HYPNOTIC, OR OPIATE DRUGS (Adult)

I. **Definition**   Alterations in the sensorium usually progressing to coma as a result of the accidental or intentional ingestion or injection of large quantities of any one of a variety of central nervous system depressants.

II. **Etiology**   Barbiturates, opiates, phenothiazine tranquilizers, and other similar agents. The agent may be taken intentionally in a suicide attempt or accidentally, as in the injection of an unusually potent "street" drug, such as heroin.

III. Clinical features

A. Symptoms

1. Alteration of consciousness is present and usually progresses rapidly to coma.

2. Respiratory depression is common, including progression to apne

3. A history from those who bring the patient to the clinic often is essential in establishing the diagnosis. It is often helpful to have the patient's pill bottles or other drug containers brought to the clinic.

B. Signs

1. Varying levels of coma are present.

2. Pupils often pin point in opiate overdose.

3. Needle tracks may be present on arms at sites of previous IV injections of heroin.

4. Spontaneous respirations often are absent.

IV. Laboratory studies   None indicated in acute situation.

V. Differential diagnosis

A. Trauma.

B. Cerebrovascular disease (including all forms of strokes).

C. Severe metabolic derangements (including diabetic ketoacidosis, hypoglycemia, and severe uremia).

VI. Treatment

A. Clear and maintain open airway.

B. Maintain respirations. Assisted ventilation by means of mouth-to-mouth respiration or an Ambu bag may be necessary.

C. Start IV infusion of dextrose in water. Give 50 ml of 50% glucose if hypoglycemia is suspected.

D. Carry out gastric lavage if drug ingestion is suspected.

E. Give naloxone HCl (Narcan), 0.5 mg, IV if opiate overdose is suggested by the history or physical findings. If no response, do *not*

give further naloxone as the drug itself in the absence of competing opiates may be a depressant.

VII. **Complications** None in acute situation.

VIII. **Consultation − referral**

A. Immediate telephone consultation for all patients.

B. Referral as soon as patient is stabilized and adequate help is available (preferably an ambulance or rescue squad).

IX. **Follow-up** Close psychiatric management if overdose is a suicide attempt.

SHOCK (Pediatric and Adult)

I. **Definition** A clinical state almost always associated with hypotension that leads to inadequate cellular perfusion and is manifested by a clinical syndrome described in **III**.

II. **Etiology**

A. **Hypovolemia** Loss of blood or other body fluid, e.g., bleeding, diarrhea, vomiting, and excessive perspiration.

B. **Cardiogenic disorders** Myocardial infarctions, arrhythmias.

C. **Sepsis** Generally from gram-negative organisms.

D. **Anaphylaxis.**

E. **Drugs** For example, barbiturates and hypotensive agents.

F. **Heat prostration.**

III. **Clinical features**

A. **Symptoms**

1. **General** Patient manifests anxiousness, confusion, and stupor.

2. **Specific** (related to etiology)

a. **Hypovolemia** Early in the sequence of events leading to hypovolemic shock the patient may be syncopal on standing because of orthostatic hypotension. Patient may have a history of severe diarrhea and vomiting or inadequate fluid intake while working outside in hot weather.

b. **Cardiogenic shock** The characteristic pain of myocardial infarction may predominate and may be accompanied by diaphoresis.

c. **Sepsis**

   (1) **Infants** Poor feeding, lethargy, and fever or hypotherm

   (2) **Adults** Fever or hypothermia, chills, lethargy, sweating (Septic shock is seen especially with urinary tract infections in the elderly or in patients with indwelling catheters.)

d. **Anaphylaxis** Insect sting or drug injection is the most common cause.

e. **Drug** Patients usually are stuporous or in coma with barbitur overdose. Hypotensive agents initially cause orthostatic hypotension.

B. **Signs**

1. **General**

   a. Hypotension. (With volume depletion initially there may be only an orthostatic fall in blood pressure.)

   b. Tachycardia.

   c. Cool, moist skin.

   d. Thready pulse.

   e. Sweating.

   f. Pallor.

   g. Decreased urine output.

2. **Specific** (related to etiology)

   a. **Hypovolemia**

      (1) **Bleeding**

         (a) **External** Usually obvious, but large quantities of blood may be sequestered in the thigh owing to fracture of the femur.

         (b) **Internal** Usually due to trauma or bleeding peptic ulcer manifested by hematemesis or coffee ground vomitus and melena.

      (2) **Dehydration** Decreased skin turgor, dry mouth, and sunken eyes.

b. **Cardiogenic shock**

   (1) Findings may be only those cited in **B.1** that are related to lowered cardiac output.

   (2) In severe shock, symptoms of congestive heart failure may be present.

c. **Sepsis** Patient usually is febrile, although elderly people, neonates, and patients with gram-negative sepsis may be afebrile or hypothermic. He may have signs related to underlying urinary tract infection, meningitis, etc.

d. **Anaphylaxis**

   (1) **Bronchospasm** Wheezes, increased expiratory phase are present.

   (2) **Urticaria or angioedema** are present sometimes.

   (3) **Laryngeal edema** Inspiratory stridor.

e. **Drug** Patients having taken barbiturates sufficient to cause shock are usually stuporous or in coma.

IV. **Laboratory studies** In the initial assessment of shock there is very little need for most laboratory tests, but if the cause is obscure, hematocrit and blood sugar determinations may be helpful. Do not wait for results before starting treatment. For later blood studies, see **VI.I.**

V. **Differential diagnosis** See **II.**

VI. **Treatment** A physician should be consulted about the treatment of all patients. Emergency measures, however, should be started *while* the physician is being contacted.

A. Call for help from other clinic personnel and notify physician.

B. Take vital signs. Start a flow sheet and evaluate vital signs every 5 minutes after IV infusion **(F)** has been started.

C. Assess the airway (as in any emergency):

   1. Remove vomitus, if present.

   2. Pull jaw forward.

   3. If laryngospasm is present (upper airway obstruction without foreign body or infection), treat patient as for anaphylactic shock.

D. Check breathing (auscultate the chest):

1. If there are wheezes, consider anaphylaxis (as well as pulmonary edema from heart failure).

·2. Assist ventilation with Ambu bag and mask if necessary.

E. Check cardiac status:

1. Palpate a major vessel.

2. Quickly auscultate the heart.

F. Start an IV infusion:

1. **Fluid** Use lactated Ringer's, normal saline solution, or other volume expander, such as Plasmanate.

2. **Rate** Run as rapidly as possible up to approximately 20–30 ml per kilogram in the first 30 minutes (except for cardiogenic shock [see **J.5**]).

G. Obtain a quick history:

1. **Underlying diseases**

   a. Heart disease.

   b. Insect allergy, medication allergy.

   c. Bleeding disorder.

   d. Diabetes mellitus.

   e. Chronic urinary tract infection.

2. **Current history**

   a. Insect sting.

   b. Drug injection or ingestion.

   c. Severe chills.

   d. Gastrointestinal symptoms (vomiting, diarrhea, and abdominal pain).

   e. Symptoms of urinary tract infection.

   f. Other symptoms.

   g. Time course.

H. Do a quick physical examination:

1. **Skin** Petechiae or purpura (occasionally associated with sepsis).

   2. **Neck**   Rigidity (meningitis).

   3. **Chest**   Wheezing, rales (anaphylaxis, pneumonia, sepsis).

   4. **Heart**   Arrhythmias.

   5. **Abdomen**

   a. Size of liver.

   b. Abdominal rigidity (peritonitis).

   c. Flank pain.

   d. Prostatic tenderness.

   e. Stool for occult blood.

   f. Vomitus for blood.

I. Draw blood for:

   1. Blood culture.

   2. Complete blood count and platelet count.

   3. Electrolytes.

   4. Blood urea nitrogen.

   5. Glucose.

   6. Future use (hold).

J. Start specific treatment

   1. **Bleeding or hypovolemia**   IV fluids have been started, which is initially sufficient and lifesaving until help can be obtained.

   2. **Anaphylaxis**   See Anaphylaxis (Pediatric and Adult), **VI.B.**

   3. **Hypoglycemia**   20 ml of 50% dextrose should be given IV, without waiting for results of laboratory tests.

   4. **Sepsis**   IV fluids should be sufficient until help can be obtained.

   5. **Cardiogenic shock**   If shock and pulmonary edema are present in a setting that suggests myocardial infarction, IV fluid should not be pushed, but an open IV line is essential in administering the drugs necessary to treat this condition after consultation.

VII. Complications

A. Complications of the **etiologic** problem.

B. Complications of shock (generally **end-organ destruction**)

    1. Brain   Ischemia, leaving neurologic deficits.

    2. Kidney   Acute tubular necrosis.

VIII. Consultation – referral   All patients require immediate consultation.

IX. Follow-up   Varies with individual patient.

SMALL OPEN WOUNDS (Pediatric and Adult)

I. Definition   Lacerations that

  A. Are *not* located on the face.

  B. Do *not* penetrate the subcutaneous tissue.

  C. Are *not* associated with functional disturbance.

  D. Have *not* been made by a grossly contaminated object.

  E. Are small and sufficiently clean so that the edges can be easily approximated using adhesives or cutaneous sutures. Approximation must be carried out without trimming tissue or placing undue tension on the suture line.

II. Etiology   Any of innumerable objects that could sever the skin.

III. Clinical features   See **I**.

IV. Laboratory studies   Culture infected wounds.

V. Treatment

  A. Wounds that do not require sutures

    1. The primary consideration is to keep the wound clean and dry:

      a. Clean with warm water and soap, making sure that dirt and foreign bodies have been removed.

      b. Cover with a loose bandage that will keep out dirt and protect the wound from trauma.

    2. If there is inflammation, the wound should be soaked and washed with soap and water for 15–20 minutes 3–4 times a day and a clean dressing applied at home each day until healing begins; then daily soaking and dressing are sufficient.

    3. Tetanus immunization status should be determined:

      a. If no previous immunization, begin series of primary immunization.

      b. If incomplete immunization, complete series of primary immunization.

      c. If no booster in 5 years, give 0.5 ml tetanus toxoid.

B. Wounds that require sutures

  1. Do not suture wounds if they are more than 6 hours old, as risk of infection increases with time.

  2. Clean the wound with warm soap and water.

  3. Irrigate the wound with sterile saline solution.

  4. Anesthetize the wound with 1−2% lidocaine (Xylocaine).

  5. Palpate or probe the wound for foreign objects, such as glass.

  6. Generally, make sutures on the extremities with 4-0 silk or nylon; on the soles of the feet a larger suture material, such as 2-0 silk, may be used.

  7. Keep the sutured wound dry and covered with a clean, dry dressing for several days, changing the dressing after the first 24 hours.

  8. Remove sutures on the basis of the location of the wound:

      a. Head and trunk: 5−7 days.

      b. Extremities: 7−10 days.

      c. Soles and palms: 10−14 days.

  9. Determine tetanus immunization status (see **A.3**).

VI. Complications

  A. Infection.

  B. Reopening of the wound.

  C. Hematoma in the wound.

VII. Consultation − referral

  A. Infected wounds.

  B. Fever or chills or other evidence of systemic infection.

  C. Facial wounds.

    D. Wounds penetrating subcutaneous tissue.

    E. Wounds associated with functional disturbance.

    F. Wounds that cannot be easily cleaned.

    G. Wounds with macerated edges that cannot be easily approximated.

VIII. Follow-up

    A. Return visit for suture removal (see **V.B.8**).

    B. Return visit for complications (describe to patient).

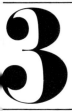

Disorders of the Skin

ACNE (Pediatric and Adult)

I. **Definition** Comedones (blackheads, whiteheads), pimples, and tender, red bumps (cysts) on the face, chest, or back, or a combination of these, usually in adolescence or early adulthood.

II. **Etiology** Increased activity of sebaceous glands, with obstruction leading to rupture of the glands. Steroids or diphenylhydantoin sodium (Dilantin) may produce eruptions in which pustules predominate and comedones are absent.

III. **Clinical features**

A. **Symptoms**

1. Lesions may be painful.

2. Stress often can be identified as a precipitating factor.

3. Psychologic consequences of the condition may be present.

B. **Signs** Increasing numbers of blackheads, whiteheads, pimples, and tender, red bumps on the face, chest, or back are seen, which may lead to pitted scars. One of these lesions may predominate or all may be present.

IV. **Laboratory studies** None.

V. **Differential diagnosis**

A. Pyoderma.

B. Drug eruptions.

VI. **Treatment**

A. **General measures**

1. Keep hands off the face. Avoid picking lesions.

2. Avoid greasy cleansing creams, oils, and cosmetics.

3. Shampoo regularly to treat seborrhea, which often accompanies acne.

4. Expect exacerbations even in the presence of treatment, especiall during menses and periods of emotional stress.

5. Eat a normal balanced diet. There is *no* need to avoid chocolate or cola.

6. Realize the value of psychological support.

B. Blackheads, whiteheads, papules, and pimples

1. General measures (see **A**).

2. Soaps and astringents

   a. For very mild acne, wash face with water and any soap 3 or 4 times a day to remove oil film.

   b. For more extensive acne, use special cleansers instead of regula soap (Fostex or Pernox). Reduce frequency of use if skin irritation occurs.

3. Drying lotions (Vanoxide or Microsyn) applied 1 or 2 times a day Reduce frequency of use if excessive dryness or irritation develop

C. Pustules and cysts

1. General measures (see **A**).

2. Soaps and astringents (see **B.2**).

3. Drying lotions (see **B.3**).

4. Antibiotic therapy for moderate to severe disease. (To avoid staining baby's teeth, do not use during pregnancy.) Consult physician before starting.

   a. Tetracycline, 250 mg 4 times a day, 1 hour before or 2 hours after meals and at bedtime for 3 weeks. Then decrease to:

   b. Tetracycline, 250 mg 2 times a day 1 hour before or 2 hours after meals until the lesions are under good control. Then decrease to:

   c. Tetracycline, 250 mg daily for several months.

   Note   In some cases tetracycline may be decreased to 250 mg every other day or discontinued completely in the summer. On the other hand some patients need a continued dosage of 250 mg 2 or 3 times a day.

   d. Tetracycline side-effects: *Candida* vaginitis, nausea, vomiting, diarrhea.

VII. **Complications**

   A. Secondary bacterial infection.

   B. Excessive dryness of skin due to overvigorous washing and use of lotion.

   C. Tetracycline side-effects.

   D. Psychologic consequences.

VIII. **Consultation — referral**

   A. Secondary bacterial infection.

   B. Resistance to therapy or sudden, persistent worsening after initial improvement.

   C. Severe psychologic stress associated with the lesions.

   D. Moderate to severe pustular acne requiring antibiotics.

IX. **Follow-up**

   A. **Tetracycline treatment**

      1. Weekly visits until the acne is under good control and the patient is taking a single daily dose.

      2. Monthly visits while patient is taking maintenance dose of tetracycline.

   B. **Nonantibiotic treatment**

      1. In 2 weeks to assess response.

      2. As needed on the basis of the severity of the lesions, the patient's compliance with the regimen, and his need for psychologic support.

ATOPIC DERMATITIS (Pediatric and Adult)

 I. **Definition**   A chronic inflammatory disease of the skin characterized by pruritus and tending to occur in patients with an allergic diathesis. Onset is commonly in infancy after age 2 months.

II. **Etiology**   Unknown. Manifestations are usually secondary to pruritus and scratching of the sensitive skin. The following may initiate and aggravate the itching and inflammation:

   A. Dry skin (cold weather).

   B. Perspiration (hot, humid weather).

   C. Certain foods (orange or tomato juice) on contact with the skin, especially in infants.

   D. Irritating clothing (wool, silk).

   E. Certain soaps, detergents, or cosmetics.

   F. Emotional stress.

III. **Clinical features**

   A. Symptoms

   1. Pruritus.

   2. Often, family history of allergic diseases (asthma, allergic rhinitis, urticaria) or atopic dermatitis.

   3. History of asthma and allergic rhinitis (about 50% of cases).

   B. Signs

   1. **Infancy**

   a. Rough, erythematous, papular, and occasionally vesicular or scaling eruption, which frequently progresses to weeping and crusting.

   b. Onset after 2 months of age.

   c. Location: Commonly on cheeks, scalp, postauricular area, neck, and extensor surface of forearms and legs; occasionally on trunk and diaper area.

   d. Fairly rapid alternation between quiescent periods and exacerbations.

   e. Frequent rubbing of involved areas by infant.

   f. In many patients, resolution of the condition by age 2.

   2. **Childhood**

   a. Less weeping and crusting, and more dry, papular, scaling eruption with hypopigmentation.

   b. Intensely pruritic and excoriated lesions.

   c. Location: Commonly on flexor surfaces of wrists and on antecubital and popliteal areas.

3. **Adolescence and adulthood**

   a. Dry, thickened skin, with accentuation of normal lines and folds. Often, hyperpigmentation.

   b. Location: Commonly on flexor areas of extremities, eyelids, back of neck, and dorsum of hands and feet.

IV. **Laboratory studies**   None.

V. **Differential diagnosis**

   A. Seborrheic dermatitis (sometimes impossible to differentiate in infancy).

   B. Fungal infections of the skin.

   C. Contact dermatitis (e.g., poison ivy).

   D. Irritant dermatitis (e.g., diaper dermatitis).

   E. Rare systemic diseases of infancy associated with an atopic dermatitis type of rash (e.g., phenylketonuria, Wiskott-Aldrich syndrome, histiocytosis X, acrodermatitis enteropathica).

VI. **Treatment**

   A. Avoidance of factors that initiate pruritus and irritate skin:

   1. Spend time outdoors in warm weather. Humidify home in winter if heating system dries air.

   2. Prevent dry skin:

      a. Minimize duration of baths.

      b. Avoid excessive exposure to soap. Use a mild soap (e.g., Neutrogena) for cleaning dirty areas.

      c. Apply agents that seal water into the skin after it is moistened by a bath or shower (e.g., Alpha-Keri, Domol, Nivea, Aquaphor, Eucerin, petrolatum).

   3. Use warm water for brief baths or showers. Hot water causes pruritus.

   4. Use soft cotton clothing and bedding. Avoid wool, starched, or rough clothing.

   5. Place a cotton pad under the bed sheets to further separate an infant from a plastic mattress.

6. Keep fingernails short.

B. Therapy of active dermatitis

1. For weeping or crusted lesions, apply soft cloth compresses of clear water at room temperature for 15 minutes 4 times a day for softening and debriding of crust and control of exudative reaction and pruritus.

2. After the acute, exudative phase has been controlled, apply a corticosteroid to the affected area:

   a. Hydrocortisone, 1%, in Eucerin cream is applied 4 to 6 times a day.

   b. The importance of frequent application of a small amount, gently massaged into the affected area, must be emphasized.

3. Use an antihistaminic (see Table 3-1) for antipruritic and sedative effect.

4. Secondary bacterial infection (beta-hemolytic streptococcal or staphylococcal) is common and must be treated before atopic dermatitis can be controlled. Consult physician.

VII. Complications

A. Secondary **bacterial infection** (beta-hemolytic streptococcal or staphylococcal).

B. Secondary **viral infection** (vaccinia or herpes simplex). Generalized vesiculopustular lesions develop, and the patient can become seriously ill.

Note   Patients with atopic dermatitis and persons with whom they have close contact should *not* be vaccinated against smallpox.

Table 3-1   Oral Dosage of Diphenhydramine (Benadryl) as an Antipruritic and Sedative

Drug Form	Body Weight	Dose	Frequency
Benadryl elixir (12.5 mg per 5 ml)[a]	8–10 kg (18–22 lb)	5.0 ml	
	10–15 kg (22–33 lb)	7.5 ml	
	15–20 kg (33–44 lb)	10.0 ml	
	20–30 kg (44–66 lb)	15.0 ml	3 or 4 times a day
or			
Benadryl capsules (25 mg per capsule)[a]	15–25 kg (33–55 lb)	1 capsule	
	Over 25 kg (over 55 lb)	2 capsules	

[a]Caution: May cause drowsiness.

III. Consultation − referral

    A. Secondary bacterial infection.

    B. Failure to respond to treatment within 2 weeks.

IX. **Follow-up**   Return visit in 1 week and periodically as needed.

DIAPER DERMATITIS

  I. **Definition**   Inflammation of the skin within the area usually covered by the diaper. It can be caused and aggravated by many factors acting separately or in combination, and a variety of morphologic changes can result.

 II. **Etiology**

    A. **Contact irritants**

       1. **Urine** (Irritation is probably caused by ammonia and other break-down products.)

          a. Diaper is not changed frequently enough.

          b. Occlusive plastic pants allow moisture and warmth to irritate and macerate skin.

       2. **Stool**

          a. Diaper is not changed frequently enough.

          b. Perineum is not cleaned thoroughly after defecation.

          c. Diarrhea.

       3. **Chemicals**   Detergents and soaps.

       4. Discharge from vulvovaginitis.

    B. **Infection**

       1. **Bacterial**   This is usually a secondary irritating colonization by a variety of organisms. Sometimes small staphylococcal furuncles are present.

       2. **Fungal**   *Candida albicans* organisms also may cause what is usually a secondary infection. It may be associated with oral candidiasis (thrush). Broad-spectrum antibiotic therapy, e.g., ampicillin, may cause candidiasis. Occasionally an infant acquires the infection through contamination of the hands of an adult with vaginal candidiasis.

      3. **Viral**   Vaccinia lesions may spread to the area of dermatitis.

   C. **Underlying skin disorder** exaggerating the effects of contact irritation and infection

      1. Seborrheic dermatitis.

      2. Atopic dermatitis.

III. Clinical features

   A. **Symptoms**

      1. Sometimes none.

      2. Pruritus.

      3. Irritability.

   B. **Signs**

      1. Erythema is present, especially on the buttocks, genitalia, and lower abdomen.

      2. Erythematous papules, vesicles, and pustules as well as superficial ulcerations are present.

      3. Affected area may be moist and exudative.

      4. During healing of moderate to severe dermatitis, skin may be dry and scaly.

      5. *Candida* characteristically produces diffuse erythema that may be moist with satellite papules and pustules outside the margin of the erythema. The patient may also have oral candidiasis.

IV. Laboratory studies   Potassium hydroxide preparation of pustule contents or scraping of affected area if candidiasis is suspected and morphology is not typical.

V. Differential diagnosis   None.

VI. Treatment

   A. **General treatment and prevention**

      1. Keep diaper area dry and free from urine and stool:

        a. Change diapers frequently.

        b. Wash contaminated area with warm water at each diaper change. Use mild, nonperfumed, nonmedicated soap sparingly to avoid irritation.

      c. Allow air to circulate under diaper:

         (1) Use only one layer of diaper pinned loosely.

         (2) Do not put plastic pants over diaper.

         (3) Expose involved areas as much as possible to air.

  2. Clean diapers well:

     a. Rinse thoroughly to remove soap.

     b. In the final rinse use a disinfectant (benzalkonium chloride [Zephiran] solution, 4 tablespoons per quart of water, or Diaparene).

B. Mild inflammation (noncandidal)

  1. Follow general hygiene (see **A**).

  2. Apply bland ointment after each diaper change, e.g., petrolatum, A and D ointment (lanolin and petrolatum), Diaparene.

C. Moderate to severe inflammation (noncandidal)

  1. Follow general hygiene (see **A**).

  2. For severe inflammation and weeping, apply aluminum acetate (Burow's) solution compresses for 20 minutes 3 times a day.

  3. If there is no weeping, apply 1% hydrocortisone cream 4 times a day.

D. Candidiasis

  1. Use good general hygiene (see **A**).

  2. Apply Nystatin (Mycostatin) cream liberally to affected area 3 times a day

    or

    Apply Mycolog cream (a combination of nystatin, steroid, and antibiotic) to affected area 2 or 3 times a day.

  3. If oral candidiasis is present or dermatitis is severe or recurrent, use Nystatin (Mycostatin) oral suspension (100,000 units per milliliter) in a dosage of 1 ml orally 4 times a day for 1 week. Drop slowly in the anterior portion of the mouth, not in the back of the throat, so that the medication is in contact with oral lesions as long as possible. It may be helpful to rub a portion of the dose on oral lesions with a cotton swab.

      4. Examine mother for candidal vaginitis if infant has recurrent candidal diaper dermatitis.

VII. Complications

    A. Spread to contiguous areas of abdomen and thighs.

    B. Severe secondary bacterial infection.

VIII. Consultation – referral   Failure to respond to treatment within 1 wee

 IX. Follow-up   Return visit in 1 week if there is no improvement.

SEBORRHEIC DERMATITIS (Pediatric and Adult)

 I. Definition   Oily, scaling condition affecting areas with large numbers of sebaceous glands.

 II. Etiology   Unknown.

III. Clinical features

    A. Symptoms

       1. Frequently, pruritus.

       2. Sometimes, no symptoms.

    B. Signs

       1. Usually, symmetric scaly eruption, often starting in scalp (cradle cap in infants).

       2. Progression to:

          a. Eyebrows.

          b. Eyelids (scales around base of eyelashes).

          c. Nasolabial and postauricular folds, external auditory canal.

          d. Presternal area.

          e. Axillae and groin.

          f. Diaper area in infants.

       3. Greasy scales, oily hair.

       4. Occasional association with acne.

       5. In infants, usually short-lived course without recurrence; in adult tendency to recur.

IV. **Laboratory studies**   Potassium hydroxide preparation is negative in pure seborrhea; perform when diagnosis is in doubt or associated *Candida* infection is suspected.

V. **Differential diagnosis**

   A. Tinea capitis or corporis.

   B. Psoriasis.

   C. Contact dermatitis.

   D. Candidiasis.

VI. **Treatment**

   A. **Adults**

      1. **Mild cases involving primarily the scalp**

         a. Use any nonprescription dandruff shampoo every 2 or 3 days (less often after symptoms subside). Lather, massage, and rinse well. Repeat sequence; leave second lather on scalp 6–10 minutes.

         b. If desired, use 2% sulfur and 2% salicylic acid cream twice a day on the skin.

      2. **Severe cases**

         a. Use one of the following tar-containing shampoos every 2 or 3 days, or as often as every day if necessary:

            (1)   Sebutone.

            (2)   Vanseb-T.

            (3)   Ionil-T.

            (4)   Pentrax.

         b. Apply 2% sulfur and 2% salicylic acid cream twice a day to affected areas.

         c. Apply a cortisone-containing lotion (1% hydrocortisone):

            (1)   Scalp: Twice a day for 10 days, then once a day for 7 days, then periodically as needed.

            (2)   Other areas: Once a day for 7–10 days, then as needed. Once the rash on the scalp is controlled, eruptions usually disappear from the face and ears.

B. Pediatric

1. Scalp

a. **Mild cases**   Use any nonprescription shampoo. Lather, mass[e] scalp with brush (soft brush for infant), and rinse well. Repe[at] sequence. Shampoo every other day until scales are gone, th[en] twice a week.

b. **Extensive or thick scaling (cradle cap)**

(1)   Use 2% sulfur and 2% salicylic acid shampoo (e.g., Sebulex). Lather, massage scalp with brush (soft brush for infant), and rinse well. Repeat sequence. Shampoo for next 2 days, then twice a week until scales are gone[.]

(2)   Use any nonprescription shampoo, with scalp massage, twice a week to prevent build-up of scales after using sulfur and salicylic acid shampoo treatment.

2. **Skin** (Oily skin with nonerythematous papules, as found on face[s] and near hairline of infants).

(1)   Wash twice a day with mild soap and water.

(2)   Do not oil skin.

(3)   Provide reassurance.

C. Erythema and scaling

1. Carry out potassium hydroxide examination of scales if the affected area is moist and in diaper or intertriginous areas, to rul[e] out candidiasis.

2. Apply 1% hydrocortisone cream 4 times a day until dermatitis clears.

VII. Complications

A. Secondary bacterial infection (usually beta-hemolytic streptococcal or staphylococcal).

B. Candidal infection, especially in intertriginous, moist areas. Infecti[on] is more likely in obese patients.

C. Contact dermatitis from medicated shampoo or lotion.

VIII. Consultation – referral

A. Secondary bacterial infection.

B. No response to treatment.

IX. **Follow-up**   Return visit in 1 week if there is no improvement.

FOLLICULITIS, FURUNCLES (BOILS), CARBUNCLES
(Pediatric and Adult)

I. **Definition**

A. **Folliculitis**   A localized infection of a hair follicle. In areas of much hair, e.g., axilla, multiple infected follicles may be present.

B. **Furuncle**   A large, deep follicular infection with one drainage point.

C. **Carbuncle**   A large coalescence of furuncles with several drainage points, most commonly occurring in the back of the neck, the back, and thighs.

II. **Etiology**   *Staphylococcus aureus.* Preceding cutaneous trauma or lesion, immunologic deficiencies, diabetes, and nasal colonization with a virulent strain all predispose to infections.

III. **Clinical features**

A. **Symptom**   Pain.

B. **Signs**

1. Lesions vary in size from erythematous papules to large nodules with one or more drainage points.

2. Lesions are extremely tender, erythematous, and surrounded by inflammation.

3. Lesions initially are firm, but centers progress to become fluctuant.

4. Regional lymphadenitis may be present.

IV. **Laboratory studies**   There is no need to culture routinely in a patient without complicating disease or recurrences.

V. **Differential diagnosis**

A. Impetigo.

B. Foreign objects, with associated infection.

C. Insect bites.

VI. Treatment

A. Folliculitis   Clean with soap and water and apply hot compresses for 20 minutes 4 times a day.

B. Furuncles and carbuncles

1. Apply hot compresses for 20 minutes 4–6 times a day until fluctuant and ready for drainage.

2. Incise and drain when fluctuant, after physician consultation.

VII. Complications

A. Usually, very few.

B. Recurrences.

C. Bacteremia with metastatic infection.

VIII. Consultation – referral

A. Carbuncles.

B. Fever.

C. Cellulitis or furuncles on the face.

IX. Follow-up

A. Folliculitis   Return visit if lesions do not clear within a week.

B. Furuncle   Return visit every other day until ready for drainage, the in 48 hours for dressing change. Further follow-up depends on size of lesion.

HERPES SIMPLEX (Pediatric and Adult)

I. Definition   A vesicular eruption of skin and mucous membranes appea ing in two distinct clinical syndromes.

A. Herpes simplex appears most often in children in its primary form and in adults in a less severe, recurrent form.

B. Herpes progenitalis appears as a primary and recurrent problem in sexually active persons.

II. Etiology   Two similar but antigenically different strains of herpesvirus hominis:

A. Type 1 (herpes simplex) usually affects skin and mucous membrane above the umbilicus.

B. **Type 2 (herpes progenitalis)** usually affects skin and mucous membranes below the umbilicus. After the primary infection, the virus remains latent in cells that are in the area of the original lesions.

III. Clinical features

A. Type 1

1. **Primary infection (acute gingivostomatitis)** appears in persons not previously infected by the virus, usually children. The initial infection may be subclinical and asymptomatic.

   a. **Symptoms**

      (1)   Soreness of the mouth and salivation.

      (2)   Fever (as high as 105° F in children).

      (3)   Malaise.

      (4)   Course of 1–3 weeks.

   b. **Signs**

      (1)   Vesicular eruption of gingival mucosa.

      (2)   Breaking of vesicles, with grayish ulcerations.

      (3)   Inflammation and swelling of gums and, sometimes, bleeding.

      (4)   Usually, enlarged, tender submandibular lymph nodes.

      (5)   Fever (as high as 105° F in children).

      (6)   Infrequently, only tonsillar lesions.

2. **Recurrence**

   a. **Symptoms**

      (1)   Burning and pain in affected area.

      (2)   Generally, no systemic symptoms unless associated with another disease.

      (3)   Reactivating factors: Stress, physical trauma, sunlight, fever.

      (4)   Course of about 1 week.

   b. **Signs**   Vesicles and ulcers usually around vermilion border of lips.

B. Type 2

1. Primary infection

   a. Symptoms

     (1)   Incubation period of 3–7 days.

     (2)   Mild to severe discomfort.

     (3)   Sometimes, prodrome of mild paresthesia or burning.

     (4)   Later, continuous vulval or penile pain, which may be severe.

     (5)   Dysuria and occasionally urinary retention.

     (6)   Tenderness of infected area.

     (7)   Sometimes, dyspareunia.

     (8)   Fever, headache, malaise.

     (9)   Course of 3–6 weeks.

   b. Signs

     (1)   Indurated papules or vesicles surrounded by erythema that often coalesce to form large ulcers.

     (2)   Location: Vulva, genitocrural folds, perianal skin, vagina and cervical mucosa in females, and urethral meatus and penis in males.

     (3)   Maceration in moist areas.

     (4)   With extensive involvement, edema is present.

     (5)   Inguinal lymphadenopathy.

     (6)   Low-grade fever.

     (7)   Sometimes, urethral discharge in males.

2. Recurrent infection

   a. Symptoms

     (1)   Symptoms are similar to those of the primary infection but usually less severe.

     (2)   Reactivation of the latent virus is related to fever, emotional disturbance, premenstrual tension.

    b. Signs

       (1) Lesions are found in the same location as the primary infection.

       (2) Signs tend to be less severe than those of the primary infection.

       (3) Early lesions are vesicles, which rupture and tend to ulcerate.

IV. Laboratory studies None. Diagnosis is made on the basis of the clinical syndrome.

V. Differential diagnosis

  A. Primary infection with herpesvirus type 1 may produce a generalized eruption that resembles chickenpox.

  B. Coxsackie and ECHO viruses cause herpangina, with papules, vesicles, and ulcers on the anterior tonsillar pillars, tonsils, soft palate, pharynx and posterior buccal mucosa. If herpes simplex lesions begin posteriorly, as they occasionally do, they may be confused with herpangina.

  C. Lesions localized to the tonsils and pharynx may be confused with pharyngitis or tonsillitis of bacterial (most commonly streptococcal), viral, or mycoplasmal origin.

VI. Treatment

  A. Type 1

    1. Primary infection

      a. General measures

        (1) Take acetaminophen (Tylenol) or aspirin for pain or fever. (See Chapter 5, Upper Respiratory Tract Infection [Pediatric and Adult], **VI.C.1** and **2** for dosage.)

        (2) Use saline solution as mouthwash or for gargling.

        (3) Apply topical anesthetic, such as Xylocaine (lidocaine) jelly, to lesions as necessary.

        (4) Isolate from certain patients (see **VII.D**).

        (5) Encourage fluid intake, especially in children, to prevent dehydration. Use bland liquids (not citrus juices or

carbonated drinks). Use straws to avoid lip, tongue, an
gum lesions.

b. **Specific measures** None.

2. **Recurrence**

a. **General measures**

(1)   Apply a local drying or soothing agent (e.g., Blistex or
Debrox) 3 or 4 times a day.

(2)   Isolate from certain patients (see **VII.D**).

b. **Specific measures** There is no established specific therapy fe
fever blister; however, 0.5% idoxuridine ointment (Stoxil) m
be used. Apply every hour for the first day, then 4 times a d

B. **Type 2**

1. **Primary infection**

a. **General measures**

(1)   Take acetaminophen or aspirin (see Chapter 5, Upper
Respiratory Tract Infection [Pediatric and Adult],
VI.C.1 and 2 for dosage).

(2)   Take sitz baths in tepid water as often as necessary.

(3)   Use a topical anesthetic, such as Nupercaine (dibucaine
HCl), if pain is intense. Generally, however, topical
anesthetics are to be avoided because of the potential
for allergic reactions.

(4)   Isolate from certain patients (see **VII.D**).

b. **Specific measures** 0.5% idoxuridine ointment (Stoxil) may
be applied to lesions every hour during first day, then 4 times
a day.

2. **Recurrence**   Same as for primary infection (**1**).

VII. **Complications**

A. Involvement of other parts of the body

1. Conjunctivitis.

2. Keratitis.

3. Generalized vesicular eruption.

    B. Secondary bacterial infection (beta-hemolytic streptococcal or staphylococcal, or both) of skin lesions.

    C. Dehydration in infants and younger children with gingivostomatitis and poor fluid intake.

    D. Spread to patients at risk of developing disseminated and severe herpes simplex. Isolate from the following:

        1. Patients with open skin lesions, e.g., burns and dermatitis.

        2. Newborns.

        3. Patients on immunosuppressive therapy.

III. Consultation – referral

    A. Conjunctivitis.

    B. Keratitis.

    C. Persistent headache and vomiting, photophobia, convulsions, or neurologic findings suggestive of encephalitis.

    D. Infection in late pregnancy because of risk to newborn, in whom fatal disseminated disease can develop.

    E. Severe primary infection (type 1 or 2).

    F. Very poor oral fluid intake (usually in infants and younger children).

    G. Secondary bacterial infection.

IX. Follow-up   Return visit in 1 week if no improvement or if any of the following develops:

    A. Eye symptoms.

    B. Secondary bacterial infection.

    C. Inadequate fluid intake.

HERPES ZOSTER (SHINGLES) (Pediatric and Adult)

I. Definition   Usually a unilateral vesicular eruption distributed along the dermatomes of infected nerve roots. It is thought to be due to reactivation of a latent viral infection.

II. Etiology

    A. Herpes zoster is caused by a virus that appears to be the same as the chickenpox virus.

B. Certain patients, particularly those with altered immune responses, have an increased tendency toward development of herpes zoster:

1. Patients with lymphomas, especially Hodgkin's disease.

2. Patients on corticosteroids.

3. Patients on other immunosuppressive agents.

4. Patients with disseminated malignancies.

III. Clinical features

A. Symptoms

1. Fever.

2. Pain, occasionally quite severe, along a dermatome. (Pain may begin as long as 3–5 days before the rash begins.) Children may not have pain.

B. Signs

1. Eruption begins with red macules; progresses sequentially to papules, vesicles, pustules, and crusts; and resolves over 1–2 we

2. Vesicles appear in clumps over the first week.

3. Involvement is unilateral.

4. Pain and eruption follow a dermatomic pattern.

5. The thoracic and cervical nerve roots are most often affected.

IV. Laboratory studies   None.

V. Differential diagnosis

A. Pain appearing before rash: Diagnosis is difficult in this situation the differential diagnosis must include any cause of pain localized the area in question. (After rash develops, the distribution and ap ance of herpes zoster are typical.)

B. Impetigo.

C. Herpes simplex.

VI. Treatment

A. General therapy

1. Take acetaminophen (Tylenol) or aspirin for fever or pain (see ter 5, Upper Respiratory Tract Infection [Pediatric and Adult] **VI.C.1** and 2 for dosage).

2. If needed, use a narcotic for pain. Consult physician.

3. Use cool water or aluminum acetate (Burow's) solution soaks for vesicles or crusts.

4. Isolate from patients listed in **II.B.**

B. Specific therapy None.

VII. **Complications**

A. Dissemination

1. In more than 50% of patients with Hodgkin's disease.

2. Rarely in patients without underlying immunologic problems.

B. Bacterial superinfection.

C. Postherpetic neuralgia (continued pain in dermatome site after rash has disappeared).

III. **Consultation – referral**

A. Any patient on steroids or other immunosuppressive drugs.

B. Coexisting Hodgkin's disease or other malignancy.

C. Symptoms persisting beyond 2 weeks.

D. Bacterial superinfection.

E. Ocular involvement.

IX. **Follow-up** Return visit if there is no improvement within 2 weeks.

IMPETIGO (Pediatric and Adult)

I. **Definition** A condition involving the superficial layers of the skin characterized by seropurulent vesicles surrounded by an erythematous base.

II. **Etiology and epidemiology**

A. Impetigo is caused by group A beta-hemolytic streptococci. Coagulase-positive staphylococci are frequently found with the streptococci. Rarely, staphylococci may be found alone.

B. It may be spread by direct contact with infected persons and possibly by insects, or it may be secondary to streptococcal infections of the upper respiratory tract.

C. Incubation period is 2–10 days.

D. The untreated patient is contagious until the lesions are healed; treatment shortens the period of contagiousness.

E. Impetigo may be a complication of insect bites, abrasions, or dermatitis.

F. Peak incidence is in late summer and early fall.

G. Impetigo is most common in infants and children.

III. Clinical features

A. Symptoms

1. Constitutional symptoms are unusual unless lesions are widespre

2. Itching is common.

B. Signs

1. Superficial vesicles are present, containing serous fluid that becomes purulent and surrounded by areas of erythema.

2. Pustules rupture, dry centrally, and form a honey-colored crust.

3. Lesions vary in size from a few millimeters to several centimeter

IV. Laboratory studies   If the diagnosis is in doubt, culture fluid from an intact vesicle or pustule or the base of a lesion after the crust is remove

V. Differential diagnosis

A. Noninfected insect bites.

B. Herpes simplex.

C. Chickenpox.

D. Other vesicular or ulcerating skin lesions.

VI. Treatment

A. Soak and then gently scrub lesions with warm water and soap three times a day to soften and remove crusts.

B. Trim fingernails to prevent further spread.

C. Use antibiotic therapy for all patients with more than a few lesions; there is some debate among authorities about the use of penicillin f treatment of patients with one or two small lesions. (Antibiotic therapy will promote healing, decreasing the period of contagiousne and therefore the spread of impetigo. It is not known whether earl treatment of streptococcal impetigo will decrease the incidence of secondary nephritis.)

1. Benzathine penicillin G (Bicillin, long-acting) (Ask whether patient is allergic to penicillin.)

   a. Children under 10 years of age: One IM injection of 600,000 units.

   b. Children over 10 years of age: One IM injection of 900,000 units.

   c. Adults: One IM injection of 1,200,000 units.

   or

2. Oral penicillin (children and adults) (Ask whether patient is allergic to penicillin.)

   a. Penicillin V, 250 mg 3 times a day for 10 days

   or

   b. Buffered penicillin G, 250,000 units 3 times a day 1 hour before or 2 hours after meals for 10 days.

   or

3. If patient is allergic to penicillin:

   a. Use erythromycin as directed in Table 3-2.

   Table 3-2   Oral Dosage of Erythromycin Suspension (200 mg per 5 ml)

Body Weight	Dose (Taken 1 Hour Before Meals)	Frequency
5−7 kg (11−15 lb)	100 mg (2.5 ml)	
7−10 kg (15−22 lb)	200 mg (5 ml)	2 times a day for 10 days
10−25 kg (22−55 lb)	400 mg (10 ml)	
25−50 kg (55−110 lb)	600 mg (15 ml)	

   or

   b. If patient weighs more than 25 kg (55 lb), use erythromycin tablets (250 mg per tablet), 500 mg (2 tablets) twice a day for 10 days taken 1 hour before meals.

   Note: If abdominal discomfort develops, divide dose in half and give 4 times a day.

D. Treat all people in close contact with patient who have impetiginous lesions as soon as possible to avoid reinfection and further spread.

VII. Complications

A. Acute glomerulonephritis may follow infection if the strain of streptococcus is nephritogenic.

B. Acute rheumatic fever is *not* a complication.

VIII. Consultation – referral

A. Failure to resolve.

B. Presence of acute glomerulonephritis in the community.

IX.. Follow-up

A. Clinic visit if no improvement within 1 week.

B. Clinic visit for persons in close contact with the patient, who have impetiginous lesions, as soon as possible.

CANDIDIASIS (Adult)

I. Definition   An infection of the skin caused by the fungus *Candida albicans.*

II. Etiology   *C. albicans.*

III. Clinical features

A. Symptoms

1. Itching.

2. Burning pain, particularly with vulvar involvement.

3. Frequent association with diabetes mellitus, particularly when diabetes is uncontrolled. Therefore, inquire about polyuria, polydipsia, and polyphagia.

4. Occasional association with use of birth control pills.

B. Signs

1. An erythematous macular rash is seen, usually involving intertriginous areas and vulva and sometimes becoming confluent with satellite lesions.

2. Vulval rash, with white, cheesy exudate, is usually associated wit candidal vaginitis. Exudate may also appear in intertriginous areas.

IV. **Laboratory studies**

    A. Potassium hydroxide preparation of the lesion is positive for *Candida.*

    B. Culture of organisms should be obtained when the diagnosis is in doubt.

    C. The level of urine or blood sugar, or both, should be measured to evaluate possible diabetes mellitus.

V. **Differential diagnosis**

    A. Seborrheic dermatitis.

    B. Other fungal skin infections.

VI. **Treatment**

    A. Coexisting diabetes   In a diabetic patient, candidiasis *cannot* be controlled or cured until the diabetes is controlled. Therefore, diabetes must be evaluated and properly managed by a physician.

    B. Intertriginous candidiasis   Apply nystatin (Mycostatin) cream twice a day.

    C. Candidal vulvovaginitis

        1. Apply aluminum acetate (Burow's) solution compresses to vulval lesions twice a day if they are moist or markedly inflamed.

        2. Use Mycostatin vaginal tablets twice a day for 10 days.

        3. Avoid contamination from gastrointestinal tract:

            a. Instruct in proper toiletry.

            b. Use Mycostatin oral tablets in recurrent cases.

VII. **Complications**   None.

VIII. **Consultation – referral**   Failure to resolve in 2 weeks.

IX. **Follow-up**   Once a week until resolution occurs.

PITYRIASIS ROSEA (Pediatric and Adult)

  I. **Definition**   A self-limited mild scaly skin eruption occurring primarily in adolescents and young adults and lasting from 3–6 weeks.

 II. **Etiology**   Unknown. Presumed to be a virus.

III. Clinical features

A. Symptoms

1. Pruritus — usually mild, sometimes intense.

2. Occasionally, mild malaise.

3. Occasionally, symptoms of a mild upper respiratory tract infecti

B. Signs

1. The herald patch is the initial lesion in most cases, but it may nc be present or may go unnoticed. It presents as a 4- to 5-cm roun or oval scaling erythematous plaque occurring anywhere on bod

2. The herald patch is followed in several days to a week by multip small 1- to 2-cm maculopapular lesions that are pale red and rou or oval with a wrinkled surface and peripheral rim of small, fine scales. These lesions occur in crops over the trunk and proximal extremities and tend to occur with their long axis oriented in th direction of the skin cleavage planes parallel to the ribs.

IV. Laboratory studies　Serologic test for syphilis to rule out secondary syphilis.

V. Differential diagnosis

A. Secondary syphilis.

B. Seborrhea.

C. Tinea versicolor.

VI. Treatment　Usually, none. Drying lotions (e.g., calamine lotion) may relieve the itching. Inform the patient that the rash will last several weeks but is self-limited.

VII. Complications　None.

VIII. Consultation — referral　None.

IX. Follow-up　Return visit as needed.

CONTACT DERMATITIS DUE TO POISON OAK, IVY
(Pediatric and Adult)

I. Definition　An acute dermatitis resulting from contact with the resin o poison oak or poison ivy.

II. **Etiology**   Most cases come from contact with the leaves of the plant; however, cases may come from digging in ground that contains the growing plant. An outbreak may also result from contact with the smoke of burning plants, unwashed contaminated clothes, dried (up-rooted) plants that still retain resin, or a pet that has had contact with the plant.

III. **Clinical features**

A. Pruritic vesicles usually appear on the extremities.

B. Early eruption may be erythematous and raised without vesicles.

C. Linear streaks of erythema or vesicles are usually seen where plant has brushed across skin.

IV. **Laboratory studies**   None.

V. **Differential diagnosis**

A. Other contact dermatitides.

B. Insect bites.

VI. **Treatment**

A. Emphasize preventive measures:

1. Instruct the patient on the appearance of the plant and how to avoid it.

2. Wash all clothes worn at the time of contact.

3. If known exposure occurs in the future, immediately wash contact area to prevent or minimize clinical symptoms.

B. Soak the affected area in saline or aluminum acetate (Burow's) solution if this can be done easily, or use cold compresses for 20 minutes 4–6 times a day. This is the mainstay of therapy.

C. Apply a drying lotion (e.g., calamine lotion) after each soak or cold compress.

D. Avoid topical lotions containing antihistaminic or benzocaine derivatives. These ingredients add nothing, and may act as allergens.

E. Use an oral antihistaminic (diphenhydramine [see Table 3-1]) for sedation and as an antipruritic in moderate to severe cases.

F. Do not use topical steroids as they are ineffective.

G. Use an oral steroid after consultation for severe cases and cases involving the eyes, face, mucous membranes, and genitalia.

VII. **Complications**   Secondary bacterial infections (see Impetigo [Pediatric and Adult]).

VIII. **Consultation – referral**

A. Widespread involvement or marked discomfort, or both.

B. Involvement of the eyes or other sensitive areas, such as oral mucous membranes and genitalia.

IX. **Follow-up**   Return visit in 3 days if there is no improvement.

SCABIES (Pediatric and Adult)

I. **Definition**   An intensely pruritic rash caused by the mite *Sarcoptes scabiei.*

II. **Etiology**

A. The initial lesion is a burrow ½–2 cm in length with a papule or vesicle at its blind end, not associated with itching. After several days, sensitivity to the mite results in severe pruritus followed by punctate excoriations from scratching and impetiginous and eczematous changes at the site of the lesion. A generalized urticarial rash may also develop.

B. The mite is transferred by personal contact, does not live long in clothing or bedding, and is found in association with poor personal hygiene and crowded living conditions.

III. **Clinical features**

A. **Symptom**   Pruritus (most severe at night).

B. **Signs**

1. The characteristic burrow appears as a thin line ½–2 cm in length ending in a papule or vesicle. Unfortunately, this sign is not seen in many patients.

2. Characteristic locations of lesions

a. Men

(1)   Interdigital folds, wrists (85% of cases).

(2) Elbows, genitalia, ankles, feet (40% of cases).

   b. Women

      (1) Palms and nipples (most frequent sites).

      (2) Other sites (see **a**).

   c. Children

      (1) Palms.

      (2) Soles of feet.

      (3) Head.

      (4) Neck.

      (5) Legs.

      (6) Buttocks.

3. Secondary changes

   a. Excoriation.

   b. Pustules and crusts of secondary bacterial infection.

   c. Eczema with weeping or scaling, or both.

IV. **Laboratory studies** Attempt to isolate the mite by scraping a burrow, papule, or vesicle and placing the specimen in mineral oil (on a slide) and examine microscopically. (Potassium hydroxide preparation [KOH] is not used because it destroys the characteristic feces.)

V. **Differential diagnosis** Scabies may take many forms and be confused with:

A. Impetigo.

B. Eczema.

C. Urticaria.

VI. **Treatment**

A. Gamma benezene hexachloride (Kwell) cream or lotion, 1%, applied after a bath to affected areas, excluding eyes, and removed in 48 hours by a bath. Repeat in 3–4 days if necessary.

B. Consultation for secondary bacterial infection.

C. Counseling on personal hygiene.

VII. **Complications**

    A. Secondary bacterial infection.

    B. Eczema.

    C. Reaction to Kwell (dermatitis).

VIII. **Consultation – referral**

    A. Failure to respond to therapy with Kwell.

    B. Absence of characteristic burrows or papules.

    C. Eczema.

    D. Secondary bacterial infection.

IX. **Follow-up**

    A. Patient should return if not cured by therapy.

    B. Other family members with skin lesions should be examined.

TINEA CORPORIS (RINGWORM OF NONHAIRY SKIN)
(Pediatric and Adult)

  I. **Definition**   Superficial fungal infection involving the trunk or limbs. (For fungal infection of the feet, see Tinea Pedis [Athlete's Foot] [Pediatric and Adult]. Refer all fungal infections of the scalp to a physician.)

 II. **Etiology**   Several different fungi.

III. **Clinical features**

    A. **Symptoms**   Condition is asymptomatic or mildly pruritic.

    B. **Signs**

       1. Erythematous, scaling patches (usually one or two) that are round or oval are seen. The lesions start small, then expand outward, with clearing of the eruption in the center of the patch and activity restricted to the border of the lesion (hence the name *ringworm*). The border of the lesion is usually raised and scaly.

       2. Lesions are most common on the face and arms.

IV. **Laboratory studies**

    A. Potassium hydroxide (KOH) preparation of scales from the active border is positive for hyphae. (Scales from the center of a lesion may be negative.)

B. Fungal culture is a more sensitive test, but takes 1–2 weeks for results and need not be done with a typical lesion.

V. **Differential diagnosis**

A. **Candidal infection**   This is usually intertriginous and redder than ringworm. It has less tendency toward central clearing, and satellite lesions are present outside the main lesion.

B. **Pityriasis rosea**   The herald patch may mimic ringworm but it is KOH-negative. Pityriasis lesions also have a more widespread distribution. Look for other pityriasis lesions elsewhere.

C. **Seborrheic dermatitis**   Lesions are usually not round or oval, and they are KOH-negative. When lesions are on the face, differentiation is very difficult. In contrast to seborrheic dermatitis, fungal infections will not clear with topical steroid treatment.

VI. **Treatment with a topical antifungal agent**   After soap and water washing and thorough drying of the lesion, apply 2 drops of 1% tolnaftate (Tinactin) solution and massage on the lesion twice a day. Two or 3 weeks are usually required; longer if thickening of the skin has occurred.

VII. **Complications**

A. Secondary bacterial infection.

B. Allergy to topical antifungal agent.

VIII. **Consultation – referral**

A. Severe or widespread infection.

B. Infection of the scalp.

C. Secondary bacterial infection.

D. Failure to respond to treatment.

IX. **Follow-up**   Return visit in 2 weeks if there is no significant improvement.

TINEA PEDIS (ATHLETE'S FOOT) (Pediatric and Adult)

I. **Definition**   A pruritic cracking and peeling eruption of the feet, especially the toe webs.

II. **Etiology**   Several different fungi.

III. Clinical features

A. Symptom   Intense itching is characteristic.

B. Signs

1. Eruptions usually start between the toes and occasionally spread to the soles or sides or even the tops of the feet.

2. Vesicles are occasionally present.

3. Toenails may be thickened, with debris under the nail.

4. Hands and groin may show evidence of fungal infection.

IV. Laboratory studies

A. Potassium hydroxide (KOH) preparation of scales or the top of vesicles for typical hyphae is optional.

B. Fungal culture may be positive when the KOH preparation is negative but need not be done with typical lesions.

V. Differential diagnosis

A. Contact dermatitis (shoe leather dye, nylon, soap, etc.).

B. Secondary syphilis.

C. Psoriasis.

D. Dyshidrosis.

E. Neurodermatitis.

F. Candidiasis.

G. Bacterial infection.

H. Reiter's disease.

VI. Treatment

A. General measures

1. Thoroughly dry interdigital areas after bathing.

2. Use absorbant cotton socks.

3. Change socks at least once a day.

B. Soaks   Soak the feet in aluminum acetate (Burow's) solution or tap water 20–30 minutes twice a day if vesicles are present. Then apply an antifungal agent (see C).

C. Antifungal agent

1. Gently massage 2 or 3 drops of 1% **tolnaftate (Tinactin) solution** onto the lesions of each foot twice a day after washing and thoroughly drying the skin.

   or

2. **Desenex (5% undecylenic acid and 20% zinc undecylenate)** is frequently effective, especially in mild cases. Sprinkle powder or apply cream between toes twice a day.

   or

3. Use **Enzactin** (triacetin) for mild cases. Apply cream twice a day.

VII. **Complications**

A. Secondary bacterial infection.

B. Allergy to topical antifungal agent.

VIII. **Consultation — referral**

A. Secondary bacterial infection.

B. No response to topical antifungal agents or worsening of condition after treatment has started.

C. Fungal infection elsewhere on the body.

IX. **Follow-up**   Return visit in 3—5 days if there is no improvement.

TINEA VERSICOLOR (Pediatric and Adult)

I. **Definition**   Benign, chronic, asymptomatic, superficial fungal infection.

II. **Etiology**   The fungus *Pityrosporon (Malassezia) furfur.*

III. **Clinical features**

A. **Symptom**   The patient shows concern about his appearance.

B. **Signs**

1. White, pink, tan, or brown macular spots, patches, or large confluent lesions are present, located mainly on the upper trunk, front and back. The lesions may extend to the abdomen and upper extremities, and less commonly to the neck and face.

2. Light scratching produces fine scales.

3. Infected areas do not tan when exposed to sunlight and appear much lighter than surrounding skin. In winter they may appear darker than surrounding areas.

IV. **Laboratory studies**   Potassium hydroxide (KOH) preparation of scales reveals large black clusters of round cells and filaments.

V. **Differential diagnosis**

A. Seborrheic dermatitis.

B. Vitiligo.

C. Pityriasis alba, if lesions are on the face.

VI. **Treatment**

A. **Counseling**   The patient should be told the following:

1. Recurrence is very common.

2. The condition is benign even without treatment.

3. Although the infection is eradicated with treatment and scaling stops, the hypopigmented areas will remain until tanned by exposure to the sun or until the surrounding tanned area fades.

B. **Selenium sulfide (Selsun) suspension**

1. Bathe or shower in the evening, scrubbing lesions with a stiff brush.

2. Apply selenium sulfide to the skin. Allow it to remain for several hours or overnight. Apply daily for 1–2 weeks.

VII. **Complications**   Irritation from selenium sulfide if it is in contact with the eyes or anogenital area.

VIII. **Consultation – referral**   No improvement after treatment and after skin color has had an opportunity to return to normal.

IX. **Follow-up**   Return visit as desired by patient.

URTICARIA (HIVES) (Pediatric and Adult)

I. **Definition**   Pruritic, red, raised plaques or welts, usually representing an allergic reaction.

II. **Etiology**   Urticaria is an allergic reaction, usually to drugs (oral and injected), foods, insect bites, inhalants, or injections. Occasionally it is due to an infection (e.g., herpes simplex, upper respiratory tract infection, tooth abscess, urinary tract infection). No cause is found in many cases.

III. Clinical features

  A. Symptoms

    1. Itching.

    2. Occasionally, stinging or paresthesia.

  B. Signs

    1. Red, raised plaques or welts with sharp borders are present usually on the trunk and extremities. They vary in number and size.

    2. Lesions usually fade in less than 12 hours, sometimes in 20–30 minutes. If lesions persist (in the same location) for more than 24 hours, the diagnosis is often erythema multiforme or multiple insect bites.

    3. The chest is clear to auscultation, and the patient is not wheezing.

IV. Laboratory studies   None.

V. Differential diagnosis

  A. Erythema multiforme.

  B. Cutaneous manifestation of anaphylaxis.

  C. Multiple insect bites.

  D. Contact dermatitis.

  E. Acute exanthem.

VI. Treatment

  A. If clinical features of anaphylaxis are present, institute immediate specific treatment (see Chapter 2, Anaphylaxis [Pediatric and Adult], VI).

  B. For widespread urticaria and intense pruritis or angioedema inject aqueous epinephrine, 1 : 1000, subcutaneously.

    1. **Pediatric dose**   0.01 ml per kg (0.005 ml per lb), maximum dose 0.3 ml.

    2. **Adult dose**   0.3–0.5 ml.

    Note   It may be necessary to repeat the dose every 1 or 2 hours for several doses.

  C. Use an antihistaminic for less severe urticaria and after injection of epinephrine (**B**).

1. Diphenhydramine (see Table 3-1)

   or

2. Chlorpheniramine maleate (Chlor-Trimeton) syrup, 2 mg per 5 m
   or tablets, 4 mg per tablet (see Table 3-3 for dosage).

Table 3-3   Oral Dosage of Chlorpheniramine Maleate (Chlor-Trimeton)

Body Weight	Dose	Frequency
10–20 kg (22–44 lb)	2.5 ml	
20–30 kg (44–66 lb)	5 ml (½ tablet)	
30–40 kg (66–88 lb)	5–7.5 ml (½ tablet)	4 times a day
Over 40 kg (over 88 lb)	5–10 ml (½–1 tablet)	

D. Search carefully for offending agent and eliminate or avoid it. Inqui
   about diet history, drug history, insect bites, etc.

E. Provide additional antipruritic effect, if necessary:

   1. Soak in a tub of cool water.

   2. Add colloidal oatmeal (Aveeno) to bath water.

VII. Complications

A. Systemic reaction to allergen, i.e., anaphylaxis or serum sickness.

B. Drowsiness secondary to antihistaminic therapy. Patients must be
   cautioned about activities requiring alertness, e.g., driving motor
   vehicles.

VIII. Consultation – referral

A. Evidence of edema of the larynx (hoarseness, inspiratory stridor).

B. Evidence of anaphylaxis (hypotension, tachycardia, paroxysmal
   coughing, severe anxiety, dyspnea, wheezing, vomiting, cyanosis).
   Treat immediately as anaphylaxis (see Chapter 2, Anaphylaxis
   [Pediatric and Adult] , **VI**).

C. Chronic or recurrent urticaria lasting more than 1 week.

IX. Follow-up

A. The patient should return in 48 hours if lesions persist or new signs
   or symptoms develop.

B. If urticaria was caused by an insect sting, he should be referred for hyposensitization.

WARTS (Pediatric and Adult)

I. **Definition**   An intradermal papilloma most frequently appearing in three distinct clinical patterns:

   A. Common warts.

   B. Plantar warts.

   C. Venereal warts.

II. **Etiology**   Human papilloma virus.

III. **Clinical features**

   A. **Common warts**

      1. **Symptoms**   Generally, none.

      2. **Signs**   Small circular skin-colored to gray-brown papillomas. These generally appear on the hand and fingers, but may appear anywhere on the skin or mucous membranes.

   B. **Plantar warts**

      1. **Symptoms**   Plantar warts may cause severe pain with walking or standing.

      2. **Signs**   These warts resemble corns or calluses, with a central nodule containing several punctate spots.

   C. **Venereal warts**

      1. **Symptoms**   Usually, none.

      2. **Signs**   Small papillomas are seen on the foreskin and penis in males (particularly those who are uncircumcised) and on the perineum and vaginal mucosa in females.

IV. **Laboratory studies**   None.

V. **Differential diagnosis**

   A. Corns, calluses.

   B. Melanoma.

VI. **Treatment**

Common warts   Apply 50—80% dichloroacetic acid every 1—2 weeks. A crust will form; this should be removed at each visit and the lesion retreated.

B. **Plantar warts**

1. **Dichloroacetic acid**   Pare down callus with scalpel and apply as directed in **A**

    or

2. **10% salicylic acid plaster**

    a. Cover the callus with plaster and bandage with tape.

    b. Remove in 5—7 days and pare down callus and wart.

    c. Treatment may be repeated, but if tenderness intervenes, wait until it subsides.

C. **Venereal warts**   Apply 25% podophyllum resin in tincture of benzoi

1. Coat area around wart with petrolatum to prevent spread of podophyllum to uninvolved area.

2. Coat warts with podophyllum mixture.

3. Allow podophyllum to remain 3—5 hours. (Use a shorter time initially, increasing the length of time with later application.)

4. Take a sitz bath after 3—5 hours.

5. Inform the patient that the lesions may be painful for several day

6. Repeat treatment at weekly intervals until warts are gone.

7. Treat any coexisting vaginitis (see guidelines in Chapter 9).

VII. **Complications**

A. Tenderness may occur around treated area.

B. Overtreatment may lead to scarring.

VIII. **Consultation — referral**

A. Large numbers of warts or large warts (which are best treated by other methods).

B. Resistance to therapy.

C. Venereal warts involving anus.

IX. **Follow-up**   As often as necessary for treatment.

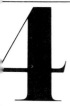

Disorders of the Eye

CONJUNCTIVITIS (Pediatric and Adult)

I. **Definition**   Inflammation of the eyelid or bulbar conjunctiva, or both.

II. **Etiology**

   A. **Bacterial infection**

      1. Pneumococcus, staphylococcus, streptococcus, Koch-Weeks bacillus, and others.

      2. Gonococcus, especially in first month of life. If the infection is contracted during birth, onset will be at age 3–5 days.

   B. **Viral infection**

      1. Associated with an upper respiratory tract infection.

      2. Conjunctivitis with epidemic sore throat, high fever, and pre-auricular and submandibular adenitis, usually due to an adenovirus.

      3. Epidemic keratoconjunctivitis, caused by adenovirus type 8.

      4. Inclusion blennorrhea, occurring in newborns and during childhood from contaminated swimming pools. This is a common disorder, and it responds to sulfonamide eye drops.

      5. Vaccinia, herpesvirus hominis type 1 (herpes simplex), herpes zoster. Lesions are usually present on the skin also.

   C. **Allergic reaction**   Conjunctivitis is often associated with seasonal allergic rhinitis, which is usually due to pollen allergy.

   D. **Foreign body or trauma.**

   E. **Chemical irritants.**

   F. **Systemic infection**

      1. Measles.

      2. Rocky Mountain spotted fever.

III. **Clinical features**

    A. **Symptoms**

        1. Mild irritation.

        2. Mild photophobia.

        3. Excessive lacrimation.

        4. Normal vision.

    B. **Signs**

        1. Injected conjunctiva.

        2. Discharge

            a. Purulent in bacterial infection.

            b. Mucopurulent in viral infection (occasionally becoming secondarily infected with bacteria).

            c. Mucoid and stringy or watery in allergic reaction.

            d. Watery when caused by a foreign body, air pollution, allergy.

        3. Sometimes, conjunctival edema.

        4. Clear cornea.

        5. Pupils are normal in size and react to light.

IV. **Laboratory studies**   Culture of exudate for gonococcus in first month of life.

V. **Differential diagnosis**

    A. **Lacrimal duct obstruction**   This is a congenital disorder seen in the first few months of life as overflow tearing and secondary bacterial infection of obstructed duct, with persistent purulent discharge.

    B. **Acute iritis** (see Table 4-1) and **iridocyclitis**.

    C. **Acute glaucoma** (see Table 4-1).

    D. **Blepharitis**.

VI. **Treatment**

    A. **Consultation** on specific cases (see **VIII**).

    B. **Allergic conjunctivitis**, if acute and mild, will respond to treatment of accompanying allergic rhinitis (see Chapter 5, Allergic Rhinitis [Pediatric and Adult]).

Table 4-1   Differential Diagnosis of Three Eye Disorders

Parameter	Acute Conjunctivitis	Acute Iritis	Acute Glaucoma
Pain	Mild discomfort	Moderate pain, with photophobia	Moderate to severe pain, with nausea and vomiting
Vision	Normal	Slightly to moderately blurred	Very blurred
Discharge	Often muco-purulent	Clear	Clear
Cornea	Clear	Clear	Cloudy
Pupil	Normal	Small and irregular	Middilated and oval
Response to light	Normal	Poor	Poor
Injection	Conjunctival only	Conjunctival and circumcorneal	Moderate to severe conjunctival and circumcorneal

C. **Mild conjunctivitis** associated with an upper respiratory tract infection is usually self-limited and need not be treated.

D. **Purulent conjunctivitis**

1. **Cool compresses** may decrease the mild discomfort that is occasionally present.

2. **Antimicrobial drops**

   a. 30% sodium sulfacetamide (Sodium Sulamyd) ophthalmic solution: Instill 1 or 2 drops in the lower conjunctival sac of the affected eye 4 times a day.

   or

   b. Neosporin ophthalmic solution (a combination of polymyxin B sulfate, neomycin sulfate, and gramicidin): Instill 1 or 2 drops in the lower conjunctival sac of the affected eye 4 times a day. **Note**   A local allergic reaction to neomycin occasionally occurs.

VII. **Complications**

A. Keratitis and scarring from gonococcus and herpes simplex.

B. Local allergic reaction to neomycin.

VIII. **Consultation — referral**

A. Any suspicion of uveitis or glaucoma (see Table 4-1).

B. Cases that might be due to the following:

    1. Gonococcus.

    2. Vaccinia, herpesvirus hominis, herpes zoster.

    3. Foreign body.

    4. Chemical irritants, particularly alkali.

C. Infants under 1 month of age.

D. No improvement in 48 hours.

IX. **Follow-up**   Return visit in 48 hours if there is no improvement.

HORDEOLUM (STYE) (Pediatric and Adult)

I. **Definition**   Localized infection of a sebaceous gland along the margin of the eyelid.

II. **Etiology**   Usually, *Staphylococcus aureus.*

III. **Clinical features**

A. **Symptoms**

    1. Some pain.

    2. No visual disturbances.

B. **Signs**

    1. Painful erythematous swelling at the margin of the eyelid.

    2. Sometimes, purulent drainage along the lid margin.

IV. **Laboratory studies**   None.

V. **Differential diagnosis**

A. Infection in a deeper gland, forming a painful swelling that drains conjunctional surface of the lid.

B. Tumors or granulomas (rare).

C. Chronic hordeolum (chalazion).

VI. **Treatment**

A. Hot compresses applied for 30 minutes every 3 hours.

B. Neosporin ophthalmic solution (a combination of polymyxin B sul neomycin sulfate, and gramicidin) in a dosage of 2 drops in the affected eye 3 times a day until drainage ceases.

VII. Complications

    A. Conjunctivitis.

    B. Cellulitis.

    C. Localized allergic reaction to neomycin.

VIII. Consultation – referral

    A. Nonpainful swelling.

    B. Failure to respond within 3 days to treatment.

IX. Follow-up

    A. As necessary for recurrence or failure to heal completely in 10 days.

    B. Return visit in 3 days if there is no improvement.

5

OTITIS EXTERNA (Pediatric and Adult)

I. **Definition**   Inflammation of the external auditory canal and auricle caused by a variety of infectious agents that may be initiated by trauma from scratching, earplugs, bobby pins, and numerous other foreign objects. Water from swimming or bathing may be absorbed by earwax (cerumen), forming a culture medium for infection.

II. **Etiology**

   A. **Bacteria**   Most commonly *Pseudomonas, Proteus,* staphylococci, and streptococci.

   B. **Fungi.**

III. **Clinical features**

   A. **Symptoms**

   1. Pain in ear.

   2. Occasionally, decrease in hearing or a sensation of obstruction in the ear.

   B. **Signs**

   1. Pain is aggravated by movement of the auricle or pressure on the tragus.

   2. The external canal may be partially occluded by edema or discharge.

   3. The external canal is usually tender when examined with an otoscope and injected or erythematous.   Exudate may be seen.

   4. The tympanic membranes may be normal, injected, or covered with flecks of exudate but does not show signs of otitis media (see Acute Purulent Otitis Media [Pediatric and Adult] and Serous Otitis Media [Pediatric and Adult], **III.B**).

   5. Preauricular or postauricular lymphadenopathy may be present.

   6. There is no swelling or pain over mastoid.

IV. **Laboratory studies**   None.

V. **Differential diagnosis**

A. **Otitis media** (see Acute Purulent Otitis Media [Pediatric and Adult] III.B). Pus may be present in the external canal, having traversed th tympanic membrane.

B. **Mastoiditis**   Swelling and pain over the mastoid area are associated with an abnormal tympanic membrane.

C. **Chronic dermatitides**   These usually are not painful but may itch chronically and may be associated with cracking and scaling of the auricle and in some cases with discharge. There is usually no pain when the auricle or tragus is moved unless it is secondarily infected Types of chronic dermatitides include:

1. Seborrhea.

2. Eczema.

3. Psoriasis.

VI. **Treatment**

A. **Prevention**

1. Fingers and instruments, including cotton swabs, should be kept out of ears. Counsel patients that the ear canal does not need cleaning.

2. Head should be kept out of water when taking a bath to avoid filling the ear canals with water and irritating dirt and soap. (Th is a relatively common cause of recurrent otitis externa in childr

3. Persistent itching of the external canal should cause the patient seek medical consultation rather than scratch with a foreign obje

B. **Specific therapy**

1. Gentle and thorough removal of debris.

2. Acetaminophen (Tylenol) or aspirin for pain (see Tables 5-9 and 5-10 for dosage).

3. Heat to ear by warm compresses, hot water bottle, or heating pa

4. Antibiotic-steroid drops into canal after thorough removal of debris. Medication will not be effective unless the canal is sufficiently clear to allow contact with inflamed tissue. Instill Cortisporin otic drops (a combination of polymyxin B sulfate, neomy cin sulfate, and hydrocortisone) in a dosage of 4 drops in the affected ear 4 times a day for one week. Patient should lie with the affected ear upward for 5 minutes after drops are instilled.

VII. **Complications**

    A. Severe otitis externa associated with:

        1. Swelling of the canal to complete closure.

        2. Severe pain.

        3. Cellulitis of the canal, auricle, and surrounding tissue.

    B. Local allergic reaction to neomycin.

VIII. **Consultation – referral**

    A. Severe otitis externa

        1. Severe pain or fever.

        2. Swelling of external canal sufficient to prevent instillation of drops and requiring a wick.

    B. Cellulitis of ear.

    C. Failure to respond to treatment in 1 week.

    D. More than one recurrence.

IX. **Follow-up** Return visit if condition persists after 1 week of treatment.

ACUTE PURULENT OTITIS MEDIA (Pediatric and Adult)

  I. **Definition** Infection in the middle ear, with accumulation of seropurulent or purulent fluid in the middle-ear cavity.

  II. **Etiology** The majority of cases are due to bacterial infection. It is not possible clinically to identify those patients with sterile exudate.

III. **Clinical features**

    A. **Symptoms**

        1. Earache.

        2. Symptoms of an upper respiratory infection.

        3. Fever.

        4. Decreased hearing.

        5. Sometimes, no symptoms.

    B. **Signs**

        1. Bulging of any portion of the tympanic membrane with accumulation of exudate in the middle-ear cavity.

2. Disappearance of the malleus (bony landmarks). The short proce
is often lost first.

3. Perforation of the tympanic membrane, resulting in the presence
of exudate in the external canal and distortion of the tympanic
membrane. (This must be distinguished from primary otitis
externa without otitis media, which is more common in the
adult.)

4. Bullae of the tympanic membrane.

5. Decreased or absent movement of the tympanic membrane with
insufflation.

Note Injection or erythema of the tympanic membrane and disappearance or distortion of the light reflex may accompany these
signs but are not alone sufficient to diagnose acute purulent otitis
media.

IV. **Laboratory studies** None.

V. **Differential diagnosis**

A. Erythema of the tympanic membrane associated with an upper
respiratory tract infection.

B. Serous otitis media.

C. Otitis externa.

VI. **Treatment** Ask whether patient is allergic to the antibiotic or antibiotics chosen.

A. **Antibiotics**

1. **Three months to 6 years of age**

a. Ampicillin suspension (see Table 5-1 for dosage)

Table 5-1 Oral Dosage of Ampicillin Suspension (250 mg per
5 ml) for Treatment of Acute Purulent Otitis Media

Body Weight	Dose	Frequency
5−7 kg (11−15 lb)	150 mg (3 ml)	
7−9 kg (15−20 lb)	200 mg (4 ml)	
9−12 kg (20−26 lb)	250 mg (5 ml)	4 times a day for 10 days
12−15 kg (26−33 lb)	350 mg (7 ml)	
Over 15 kg (over 33 lb)	500 mg (10 ml)	

or

b. Benzathine penicillin G (Bicillin) and sulfisoxazole (Gantrisin) suspension (see Tables 5-2 and 5-3 for dosage)

or

c. Penicillin V, 250 mg 4 times a day for 10 days, and sulfisoxazole suspension (see Table 5-3 for dosage).

or

d. If patient is allergic to penicillin, erythromycin and sulfisoxazole (see Tables 3-2 and 5-3 for dosages).

Table 5-2   Intramuscular Dosage of Benzathine Penicillin G (Bicillin) for Treatment of Acute Purulent Otitis Media

Age	Dose (units)	Frequency
Under 6 months	300,000	1 injection
6 months–6 years	600,000	

Table 5-3   Oral Dosage of Sulfisoxazole (Gantrisin) Suspension (500 mg per 5 ml)

Body Weight	Initial Dose Given in Clinic	Subsequent Doses	Frequency
5–7 kg (11–15 lb)	500 mg (5 ml)	250 mg (2.5 ml)	
7–9 kg (15–20 lb)	600 mg (6 ml)	300 mg (3 ml)	
9–12 kg (20–26 lb)	800 mg (8 ml)	400 mg (4 ml)	
12–15 kg (26–33 lb)	1000 mg (10 ml)	500 mg (5 ml)	
15–18 kg (33–40 lb)	1200 mg (12 ml)	600 mg (6 ml)	4 times a day for 10 days
18–22 kg (40–48 lb)	1500 mg (15 ml)	750 mg (7.5 ml)	
22–25 kg (48–55 lb)	1800 mg (18 ml)	900 mg (9 ml)	
Over 25 kg (over 55 lb)	2000 mg (20 ml)	1000 mg (10 ml)	

2. Over 6 years of age

a. Penicillin V, 250 mg 4 times a day for 10 days

or

b. Benzathine penicillin G (Bicillin) (see Table 5-4 for dosage)

Table 5-4   Intramuscular Dosage of Benzathine Penicillin G (Bicillin) for Treatment of Acute Purulent Otitis Media

Age	Dose (units)	Frequency
Children 6–10 years	600,000	
Children over 10 years	900,000	1 injection
Adults	1,200,000	

or

c. If patient is allergic to penicillin: Erythromycin tablets (250 per tablet), 500 mg (2 tablets) twice a day for 10 days taken 1 hour before meals. **Note** If abdominal discomfort develops divide dose in half and give 4 times a day.

B. **Decongestants and antihistaminic-decongestant combinations**

Note   The efficiency of these medications for the treatment of purulent otitis media has not been proved. If patient compliance with oral medication is a concern, limiting the regimen to one medication namely, the antibiotic, may be wise.

1. **Children under 12 years of age**

   a. Oral decongestant (pseudoephedrine HCl; for dosage, see Table 5-5) for mucosal inflammation and edema associated with an upper respiratory tract infection causing eustachian tube obstruction

Table 5-5   Oral Dosage of Pseudoephedrine HCl (Sudafed) Syrup (30 mg per 5 ml) for Treatment of Acute Purulent Otitis Media

Age	Dose[a]	Frequency
6 months–2 years	2.5 ml	
2–6 years	5.0 ml	3 or 4 times a day for 3 weeks
Over 6 years	7.5 ml	

[a]Dose should be decreased if side-effects (e.g., hyperactivity, irritability insomnia) occur.

or

   b. Oral antihistaminic-decongestant combination (Dimetapp; for dosage see Table 5-6) for mucosal inflammation and edema associated with allergic rhinitis (which may be complicated by an upper respiratory tract infection) causing eustachian tube obstruction.

Table 5-6   Oral Dosage of Brompheniramine-Phenylephrine-Phenylpropanolamine (Dimetapp) Elixir

Age	Dose	Frequency
6 months–2 years	2.5 ml	
2–4 years	4.0 ml	3 or 4 times a day for 3 weeks
4–12 years	5.0 ml	

2. **Adults and children over 12 years of age**

   a. Oral decongestant for mucosal inflammation and edema associated with an upper respiratory tract infection causing eustachian tube obstruction. Give pseudoephedrine HCl (Sudafed) tablets (60 mg per tablet) in a dosage of 1 tablet 3 or 4 times a day for 3 weeks.

   or

   b. Oral antihistaminic-decongestant combination for mucosal inflammation and edema associated with allergic rhinitis (which may be complicated by an upper respiratory tract infection) causing eustachian tube obstruction:

   (1)   Brompheniramine-phenylephrine-phenylpropanolamine (Dimetapp Extentabs) in a dosage of 1 Extentab 2 or 3 times a day for 3 weeks

      or

   (2)   Triprolidine HCl and pseudoephedrine HCl (Actifed) tablets in a dosage of 1 tablet 3 times a day for 3 weeks

   and/or

   c. Xylometazoline HCl (Otrivin) 0.1% nasal spray: One spray followed in 5–10 minutes by a second spray; repeat sequence every 6 hours for 2 weeks.

II. **Complications**

   A. Serous otitis media.

   B. Persistent purulent otitis media.

   C. Mastoiditis.

   D. Extension into the central nervous system, leading to meningitis or brain abscess.

   E. Chronic otitis media with perforation of the tympanic membrane.

    F. Cholesteatoma formation associated with chronic otitis media and marginal or pars flaccida perforation.

VIII. **Consultation — referral**

    A. Infants under 3 months of age.

    B. Severe pain.

    C. Failure to improve symptomatically in 48 hours.

    D. Signs of meningitis, such as:

        1. Lethargy.

        2. Extreme irritability.

        3. Bulging fontanel.

        4. Stiff neck.

    E. Persistent purulent otitis media despite adequate course of antibiotics.

    F. More than two episodes of purulent otitis media.

        1. Child: In 1 year.

        2. Adult: Over any period of time.

    G. Suspicion of mastoiditis: Pain, tenderness, or edema in the postauricular area in older children and adults.

    H. Chronic otitis media with persistent intermittent drainage through perforation of the tympanic membrane.

  IX. **Follow-up**   Examination in 3 weeks.

SEROUS OTITIS MEDIA (Pediatric and Adult)

  I. **Definition**   Accumulation of a bacteriologically sterile, nonpurulent effusion in the middle-ear cavity.

  II. **Etiology**

    A. Eustachian tube obstruction with subsequent formation of an effusion in the middle-ear cavity. The causes of eustachian tube obstruction include:

        1. Enlarged adenoids.

        2. Upper respiratory tract infection with mucosal edema.

      3. Allergic rhinitis with mucosal edema.

      4. Cleft palate.

      5. Deviated nasal septum.

      6. Nasopharyngeal tumor in adults.

  B. A complication of purulent otitis media.

  C. Possibly, active secretion by the mucosa of the middle-ear cavity in an allergic patient.

III. Clinical features

A. Symptoms

    1. Hearing loss.

    2. Feeling of fullness in the ear.

    3. Snapping sensation when swallowing, yawning, or blowing the nose.

    4. Symptoms associated with the disorders listed in **II.A** (e.g., chronic snoring associated with enlarged adenoids).

    5. Occasionally, no symptoms, especially if chronic.

B. Signs

    1. Clear or transparent yellowish fluid (early) or bluish gray fluid (long-standing) with or without air bubbles behind the tympanic membrane associated with:

      a. Retraction of the tympanic membrane.

      b. Prominence of the malleus, especially the short process, with an abnormally horizontal handle of the malleus drawn inward.

      c. Decreased or absent movement of the tympanic membrane with insufflation. Occasionally, only outward movement with negative pressure is seen.

    Note Injection or erythema of the tympanic membrane and disappearance or distortion of the light reflex, as seen in an upper respiratory tract infection or allergic rhinitis may accompany these signs but are not alone sufficient to diagnose serous otitis media.

    2. Signs associated with the disorders listed in **II.A** (e.g., mouth-breathing associated with enlarged adenoids).

    3. Decreased hearing.

IV. Laboratory studies None.

V. Differential diagnosis

  A. Acute purulent otitis media.

  B. Chronic otitis media.

  C. Retraction or erythema, or both, of the tympanic membrane without serous effusion, as seen in an upper respiratory tract infection or allergic rhinitis.

  D. Normal retracted appearance of the tympanic membrane of the very young infant.

  E. Symptoms of eustachian tube obstruction alone with a normal tympanic membrane.

  F. Hearing loss due to other causes.

  G. Meniere's disease.

VI. Treatment

  A. Children under 12 years of age

    1. See Acute Purulent Otitis Media (Pediatric and Adult), **VI.B.1.**

    2. If condition is not resolved after 3 weeks of therapy in **1**, continue the same therapy for 2 more weeks (except in infants under 3 months of age, who should be referred) and add xylometazolin (Otrivin) (see Table 5-7).

Table 5-7 Pediatric Dosage of 0.05% Xylometazoline (Otrivin) Nasal Solution

Age	Dose (in Each Nostril)	Frequency
3–6 months	1 drop	Every 6 hours
6 months–2 years	2 drops	Every 4 hours while awake
2–12 years	3 drops	Every 4 hours while awake

    3. If condition is not resolved after therapy in **2**, refer patient.

  B. Adults and children over 12 years of age

    1. See Acute Purulent Otitis Media (Pediatric and Adult), **VI.B.2.**

    2. If condition is not resolved after 3 weeks of therapy in **1**, continue the same therapy for 2 more weeks and add 0.1% xylometazoline nasal spray, one spray followed in 5—10 minutes by a second spray; repeat sequence every 6 hours.

    3. If condition is not resolved after therapy in **2**, refer patient.

VII. Complications

    A. Chronic serous otitis media causing:

        1. Adhesive otitis media with permanent conductive hearing loss.

        2. Decreased hearing with increased risk of:

            a. Defective speech development.

            b. School failure.

    B. Acute purulent otitis media.

    C. Cholesteatoma from chronic severe retraction of pars flaccida.

VIII. Consultation — referral

    A. Failure to respond to treatment. (Continue oral and nose-drop therapy until consultant appointment.)

    B. Under 3 months of age, failure to resolve after 3 weeks.

    C. More than two episodes in 1 year.

IX. Follow-up

    A. Have the patient return after 3 weeks of therapy.

    B. If the condition has not resolved after 3 weeks of therapy, schedule a follow-up visit for 2 weeks later.

    C. Always follow the patient *until resolution occurs* to avoid complications.

EPISTAXIS (Pediatric and Adult)

I. Definition   The spontaneous discharge of blood from the nares.

II. Etiology

    A. Spontaneous rupture of a blood vessel in the nose (usually the anterior septum), occurring most frequently in children and in the elderly.

    B. Higher incidence in winter, when heating causes drying and cracking of nasal mucosa.

    C. Trauma from a direct blow to the nose.

    D. Picking of dry, crusted nostrils.

    E. Rarely, hypertension.

    F. Rarely, a bleeding disorder.

III. Clinical features

    A. Symptoms   Usually none other than the awareness of blood dribbling down the posterior nasopharynx as well as external bleeding.

    B. Signs

        1. Bleeding from the nares and down the posterior nasopharynx.

        2. Localized bleeding point: This may or may not be seen in the anterior nasal septum.

        3. Usually, normal blood pressure.

        4. Usually, no orthostatic fall in blood pressure.

        5. Usually, no evidence of bleeding or clotting disorder, e.g., bruises, petechiae.

IV. Laboratory studies

    A. Generally, none.

    B. Hematocrit, if history indicates significant bleeding.

V. Differential diagnosis   None.

VI. Treatment

    A. Acute bleeding

        1. Keep the patient in an erect sitting position with his head tilted forward to prevent blood from going down the posterior nasopharynx.

        2. To decrease venous pressure, try to keep children from crying.

        3. With thumb and forefinger, apply continuous external compression on both sides of the nose for 15 minutes.

    B. Prevention

        1. Discourage picking of the nose.

    2. Increase the humidity in the home, especially in sleeping areas, by means of a humidifier or pot of water on a heater.

    3. Rub petrolatum over the nasal septum twice a day when dry or crusted.

VII. Complications   Anemia, if bleeding is excessive or frequent.

VIII. Consultation – referral

  A. Bleeding not controlled by 15 minutes of compression.

  B. Evidence of massive bleeding.

  C. Recurrent bleeding within first hour.

  D. Second episode within a week.

  E. Bleeding from the posterior nasopharynx. (Usually this cannot be controlled by the measures described in **VI.A.**)

IX. Follow-up   As needed for recurrent episodes.

ALLERGIC RHINITIS (Pediatric and Adult)

I. Definition   An allergic disease affecting the nasal mucosa and often the conjunctiva. It may be seasonal or perennial (nonseasonal).

II. Etiology

  A. Seasonal

    1. Pollens that depend on wind for cross-pollination. In the eastern United States the following are the most common causes (pollination time may vary by several months depending on location):

      a. Ragweed: August–October.

      b. Grasses: May–July.

      c. Trees: April–July.

      d. Combinations of **a, b,** and **c.**

  B. Perennial

    1. House dust.

    2. Feathers.

    3. Mold spores.

    4. Animal dander.

5. Foods: There is disagreement about the role of food in causing isolated allergic rhinitis. Most authorities believe that if foods ar causative, other signs of hypersensitivity occur with allergic rhini (e.g., urticaria, asthma, gastrointestinal symptoms).

C. **Perennial with seasonal exacerbations.**

D. **Aggravating factors**

1. Tobacco smoke.

2. Air pollutants.

3. Sudden temperature changes.

III. **Clinical features**

A. **Symptoms**   Onset is usually in childhood and young adulthood, wit symptoms decreasing with age. A family history of allergic diseases is common. Symptoms of seasonal allergic rhinitis tend to occur th same time each year and are frequently more severe than those of the perennial form.

1. Sneezing.

2. Nasal itching.

3. Watery rhinnorhea.

4. Nasal stuffiness.

5. Occasionally, other symptoms, including the following:

a. Itching of the eyes, palate, and throat.

b. Snoring and sniffing.

c. Increased tearing and photophobia.

d. Nonproductive cough from irritation of posterior pharyngeal secretions.

e. Fatigue, irritability, anorexia.

B. **Signs**

1. Clear, thin nasal discharge.

2. Pale, edematous nasal mucosa.

3. Enlarged nasal turbinates.

4. "Allergic salute": Rubbing of the nose upward and outward (see especially in children).

5. Mouth-breathing.

6. Conjunctival injection and edema. Occasionally granular, erythematous conjunctivae and swollen eyelids with extra lines and dark semicircles (allergic "shiners") under the eyes.

7. Allergic facies with perennial allergic rhinitis

   a. Mouth-breathing.

   b. Prominent maxilla, high arched palate.

   c. Dull expression.

   d. Broad midsection of nose, with horizontal crease across lower portion.

IV. **Laboratory studies**   Wright's or Hansel's stain of smear of nasal secretions may reveal eosinophils, but usually is not needed to make a diagnosis.

V. **Differential diagnosis**

   A. **Seasonal**

      1. Upper respiratory tract infection.

      2. Infectious conjunctivitis.

   B. **Perennial**

      1. Recurrent upper respiratory tract infections.

      2. Vasomotor rhinitis (of unknown cause, noninfectious, nonseasonal, and nonallergic).

      3. Deviated nasal septum.

      4. Side-effect of medications

         a. Reserpine.

         b. Vasoconstricting nose drops.

      5. Chronic sinusitis.

VI. **Treatment**

   A. **Identification and avoidance of the offending antigen**   Apply the following measures *if appropriate* for the individual patient:

      1. **Seasonal**

         a. Avoid areas of heavy concentration of ragweed, trees, or grass during pollinating seasons.

b. Sleep with bedroom windows closed during the appropriate pollinating season.

c. Use an air conditioner with an electrostatic precipitating filter to avoid pollen.

2. **Perennial**

a. Create a dust-free bedroom (patients who must do their own cleaning should use a mouth-and-nose mask):

   (1) Remove everything from the room, including floor coverings, curtains, drapes, and closet contents.

   (2) Clean the room thoroughly — walls, woodwork, ceiling, floor, and closet. Wax the floor.

   (3) Scrub the bed frame and metal springs.

   (4) Cover the mattress, box spring, and pillows with plastic dust-proof covers.

   (5) Make sure the room contains a minimum of furniture, washable rugs, and curtains. Avoid bed pads, heavy rugs, drapes, upholstered furniture, toys, and knickknacks.

   (6) Clean the room at least once a week using a vacuum cleaner, damp cloth, or oil mop. Do not use a broom or duster.

   (7) Keep bedroom windows and doors closed. If hot-air heating is used, cover vents with course muslin and change frequently. Change furnace air filter twice a year.

b. Vacuum stuffed furniture and rugs frequently.

c. Remove pets (dogs, cats, birds) from the house.

d. Avoid damp and dusty places (attics, basements, closets, storerooms).

e. Avoid stuffed toys, if patient is dust-sensitive.

f. Use an air conditioner with an electrostatic precipitating filter to avoid dust.

B. **Antihistaminic**   The goal of therapy is to achieve symptomatic relief with a minimum of side-effects, e.g., drowsiness, nervousness, dry mouth. Therefore, manipulation of dosage within the prescribed ranges may be necessary. Medication should be taken for several days to weeks at a time during symptomatic periods; since antihistaminics do not antagonize released histamine but only prevent further release, intermittent single-dose usage will not be as effective in controlling symptoms.

1. Use chlorpheniramine (Chlor-Trimeton) syrup as an antihistaminic (see Table 3-3)

    or

2. Use an antihistamine-decongestant combination (Dimetapp) (for dosage see Table 5-6 if under 12 years and Acute Purulent Otitis Media [Pediatric and Adult], **VI.B.2.b.(1)** or **(2)** if over 12 years).

VII. Complications

A. Eustachian tube obstruction causing serous otitis media.

B. Sinus orifice obstruction causing sinusitis.

C. Nasal or sinus polyps from long-standing perennial allergic rhinitis.

D. Dental malocclusion problems from maxillary deformity associated with chronic nasal obstruction.

E. Drowsiness from antihistaminic therapy.

VIII. Consultation — referral

A. Failure to respond to treatment.

B. Considerations for immunotherapy (hyposensitization)

1. Severe or prolonged periods of symptoms not controlled by treatment measures described earlier.

2. Inability to tolerate antihistaminics and more than mild symptoms.

3. Patients requiring almost daily medication for perennial allergic rhinitis.

IX. Follow-up   Return visit in 1 week, and periodically as needed.

PHARYNGITIS (SORE THROAT) (Pediatric and Adult)

I. Definition   Inflammation of the pharynx or tonsils, or both.

II. Etiology

A. Usually nonbacterial (presumed to be viral).

B. Group A beta-hemolytic streptococci.

C. Much less commonly, *Mycoplasma pneumoniae* and *Corynebacteriu* *diphtheriae.*

III. Clinical features   It is *not* possible to determine the etiology of phary gitis by clinical features alone. Although Table 5-8 may be helpful, a throat culture is needed to definitely establish whether or not pharyn gitis is due to group A beta-hemolytic streptococci.

IV. Laboratory studies

A. Throat culture of patient for group A beta-hemolytic streptococci.

Table 5-8   Findings in Pharyngitis Suggestive of Streptococcal Etiology

Clinical Feature	Very Suggestive	Moderately Suggestive	Questionably Suggestive	Unusual
Tender anterior cervical lymph nodes	All ages			
Household contact	All ages			
Scarletina-form rash	School age Adults			Infants
Excoriated nares	Infants			School a Adults
Tonsillar exudate	Adults	School age	Infants	
High fever		All ages		
Occurrence during respiratory infection season		All ages		
Acute onset		School age Adults		Infants
Sore throat		School age Adults		Infants
Abdominal pain		Infants School age		Adults
Rhinorrhea		Infants		School a Adults
Enlarged anterior cervical lymph nodes		Infants	School age Adults	
Red throat			All ages	
Hoarseness				All ages
Cough				All ages

Modified from L. A. Wannamaker, *Am. J. Dis. Child.* 124:357, 1972.

   B. Throat culture of all household contacts, ideally two days after instituting treatment for streptococcal pharyngitis in original case.

   C. White blood cell and differential counts and heterophile antibody determination in suspected cases of infectious mononucleosis (see Chapter 16, Infectious Mononucleosis [Pediatric and Adult]).

V. Differential diagnosis

   A. Infectious mononucleosis.

   B. Influenza.

   C. Stomatitis (e.g., herpetic).

VI. Treatment

   A. General measures for pharyngitis of any etiology:

   1. Acetaminophen or aspirin for high fever (see Upper Respiratory Tract Infection [Common Cold] [Pediatric and Adult], **VI.C.1** and 2 for dosage).

   2. Warm saline gargle for older children and adults.

   3. Increased fluid intake.

   B. Antibiotics for streptococcal pharyngitis   Ask whether patient is allergic to penicillin. **Note** Tetracyclines and sulfonamides should not be used for the treatment of streptococcal pharyngitis.

   1. Benzathine penicillin G (Bicillin)   (Mixtures containing shorter acting penicillins should not be substituted.)

   a. Children under 10 years of age: One IM injection of 600,000 units.

   b. Children over 10 years of age: One IM injection of 900,000 units.

   c. Adults: One IM injection of 1,200,000 units.

   or

   2. Oral penicillin   This method of therapy depends on the cooperation of the patient for 10 days. Therefore IM benzathine penicillin G is the method of choice. If oral penicillin is selected, however, specific counseling outlining the need for the ten full days of therapy to eradicate the infection and prevent rheumatic fever should be stressed.

    a. Penicillin V, 250 mg 3 times a day for 10 days

     or

    b. Buffered penicillin G, 250,000 units 3 times a day 1 hour before or 2 hours after meals for 10 days.

  or

  3. If patient is allergic to penicillin:

    a. Erythromycin suspension (see Table 3-2 for dosage)

     or

    b. If patient is over 25 kg (50 lb), erythromycin tablets (250 mg per tablet) in a dosage of 500 mg (2 tablets) twice a day for 10 days taken 1 hour before meals.

    Note   If abdominal discomfort develops, divide dose in half and give 4 times a day.

VII. Complications of streptococcal pharyngitis

A. Rheumatic fever.

B. Cervical lymphadenitis, particularly in infants.

C. Otitis media, particularly in children.

D. Peritonsillar abscess in older children and adults.

E. Retropharyngeal abscess in younger children.

F. Sinusitis.

G. Acute glomerulonephritis.

VIII. Consultation – referral

A. Cervical adenitis of 3 cm in diameter or greater.

B. Peritonsillar abscess   Consider when the following are present:

  1. Asymmetrical swelling of tonsils, tonsillar fossae, and overlying soft palate. Uvula shifted to opposite side.

  2. Fever persisting 4 days after treatment for streptococcal pharyngitis was started.

  3. Trismus, difficulty swallowing, and feeling of fullness in throat.

  4. Extreme enlargement of tonsils.

C. **Prolonged toxic course.**

D. **Retropharyngeal abscess** Consider in infant when the following are present:

1. Difficulty in swallowing.

2. Persistent high fever.

3. Hyperextended head, with difficulty in breathing.

4. Forward bulge in the posterior pharyngeal wall.

E. **Membrane on pharynx** suggesting diphtheria.

IX. **Follow-up**

A. Throat culture of all household contacts, ideally 2 days after instituting treatment for streptococcal pharyngitis in original case.

B. Because of possible noncompliance with treatment regimen, repeat throat culture 3–5 days after completion of course of oral penicillin. A repeat throat culture is *not* necessary if IM benzathine penicillin G (Bicillin) is used.

ORAL CANDIDIASIS (THRUSH) (Pediatric)

I. **Definition** Superficial fungal infection of the oral cavity in infants.

II. **Etiology** The causative organism is *Candida albicans,* which is usually acquired from the following sources:

A. Mother's vagina during birth.

B. Other infants, by contamination of caretaker's hands or objects shared by babies.

C. Adult with vaginal candidiasis, through contamination of her hands.

D. Patient's own candidal diaper dermatitis.

E. Oral broad-spectrum antibiotic therapy (e.g., ampicillin), as a side-effect.

III. **Clinical features**

A. **Symptoms**

1. Often none.

2. With extensive involvement, pain during feeding and swallowing.

B. Signs

1. White, irregularly shaped plaques appear on the buccal mucosa, lips, palate, and gums. They may produce a confluent white coating on the tongue.

2. Lesions are removable, leaving an inflamed base.

3. The patient may have candidal diaper dermatitis (moist, red, occasionally scaling rash with a sharp border and satellite red papules or pustules).

IV. Laboratory studies   Potassium hydroxide preparation of scrapings of lesions reveals budding yeast with or without hyphae. This study usually is not needed when typical lesions are present.

V. Differential diagnosis   Milk or food particles remaining in the mouth of the patient.

VI. Treatment

A. Control of source of infection

1. Wash hands thoroughly between handling of different infants in newborn nursery and before handling any baby.

2. Do not have infants share clothing, pacifiers, nipples, etc.

3. Examine and treat contact with vaginitis.

4. Treat candidal diaper dermatitis (see Chapter 3, Diaper Dermatitis).

B. Oral antifungal therapy   Use nystatin (Mycostatin) oral suspension (100,000 units per milliliter) in a dosage of 1 ml orally 4 times a day for 1 week. Drop slowly in anterior portion of mouth, not in back of throat, so that medication is in contact with the lesions for as long as possible. It may be helpful to rub a portion of the dose on the lesions with a cotton swab. This oral antifungal treatment may be repeated for another week if marked improvement does not occur.

VII. Complications

A. Feeding problems due to pain.

B. Candidal diaper dermatitis or perioral dermatitis.

C. Spread of infection to other infants in nursery or home.

VIII. **Consultation − referral**

    A. Failure to respond to 2 weeks of therapy.

    B. Failure to thrive.

IX. **Follow-up**   Return visit in 1 week if the infection is not markedly improved.

BACTERIAL SINUSITIS (Adult)

  I. **Definition**   Inflammation of the mucous membrane lining of the paranasal sinuses due to bacterial infection, causing obstruction of normal sinus discharge. In chronic recurrent disease, allergens or irritants such as smoke may initiate symptoms.

 II. **Etiology**

    A. Group A beta-hemolytic streptococci.

    B. *Hemophilus influenzae.*

    C. Hemolytic *Staphylococcus aureus.*

    D. Pneumococcus.

III. **Clinical features**

    A. **Symptoms**

       1. Mucopurulent nasal discharge and persistent postnasal drip.

       2. Choking cough at night, often appearing after a recent upper respiratory tract infection (URI).

       3. General malaise.

       4. An ache or pressure behind the eyes.

       5. Toothache-like pain.

       6. Headache (often worse at night and early morning).

    B. **Signs**

       1. Yellow mucopurulent nasal discharge.

       2. Tenderness over the involved sinus.

       3. Cellulitis in area overlying the involved sinus.

       4. Periorbital cellulitis.

      5. Edematous, hyperemic inferior turbinates.

      6. Usually, fever (101° F or higher).

IV. Laboratory and other studies

    A. X-ray (only on physician's orders).

    B. Nasopharyngeal culture.

V. Differential diagnosis

    A. Nonbacterial sinusitis.

    B. Undifferentiated URI.

    C. Persistent rhinitis due to allergy.

VI. Treatment

    A. For drainage (see Acute Purulent Otitis Media [Pediatric and Adult] VI.B.2)

      1. Decongestants.

      2. Decongestant-antihistaminic combination.

      3. Nasal spray: xylometazoline HCl (Otrivin).

    B. For fever and pain Aspirin, 1 or 2 tablets (325 mg per tablet), orally every 4–6 hours.

    C. For infection Antibiotics (telephone consultation with physician is required)

      1. Ampicillin, 500 mg orally every 6 hours for 10 days if not allergic to penicillin.

      2. Erythromycin, 250 mg orally every 6 hours for 10 days if not allergic to penicillin.

VII. Complications Complications are infrequent, but serious.

    A. Abscess.

    B. Osteomyelitis.

    C. Spread to the central nervous system.

VIII. Consultation – referral

    A. All acutely and severely ill patients.

    B. Chronic or recurrent illness.

  C. Any indication of involvement of the orbit or central nervous sys-
     tem.

IX. **Follow-up**   Have patient call in 2 or 3 days if there is no improvement.

NONBACTERIAL SINUSITIS (Adult)

  I. **Definition**   Inflammation of the mucous membrane lining the paranasal
     sinuses due to viral, allergic, vasomotor, or other nonbacterial causes,
     producing obstruction of normal sinus discharge.

 II. **Etiology**

     A. Numerous viruses, pollens, and other allergens.

     B. Vasomotor instability secondary to cold or emotional factors, or
        both.

III. **Clinical features**

     A. **Symptoms**

        1. Clear, nonpurulent nasal discharge.

        2. Nocturnal postnasal drip with resultant cough.

        3. Pain in the area of the involved sinuses that is usually appreciated
           as a sensation of pressure or fullness.

        4. Minimal or no generalized symptoms such as malaise or myalgia.

        5. Headache.

        6. Simulation of a toothache in some cases of maxillary sinusitis.

     B. **Signs**

        1. Clear nasal discharge.

        2. Edema and hyperemia of the nasal mucosa.

        3. Tenderness over the involved sinus.

        4. No cellulitis of the area over the involved sinus.

        5. No fever or temperature less than $101°$ F.

 IV. **Laboratory studies**   None.

  V. **Differential diagnosis**

     A. Bacterial sinusitis.

B. Uncomplicated upper respiratory tract infection (URI).

C. Allergic rhinitis.

D. Dental abscess.

VI. Treatment

A. **Nasal congestion**   In sinusitis alone and that associated with viral upper respiratory infection the use of decongestants or antihistamir or both, is usually sufficient to decrease edema and discomfort. Us the following (see Acute Purulent Otitis Media [Pediatric and Adul VI.B.2):

1. Decongestants.

2. Antihistaminic-decongestant combination.

3. Nasal spray.

B. **Pain**   Aspirin, 600 mg orally every 4–6 hours for fever and pain.

VII. Complications   Bacterial sinusitis.

VIII. Consultation — referral

A. Chronic or recurrent illness.

IX. Follow-up   Telephone call in 2 or 3 days if no improvement.

UPPER RESPIRATORY TRACT INFECTION (COMMON COLD)
(Pediatric and Adult)

I. **Definition**   An acute infection of the upper respiratory tract lasting several days.

II. **Etiology**   Numerous viruses.

III. **Clinical features**

A. **Symptoms**

1. General malaise.

2. Nasal stuffiness, nasal discharge, sneezing, cough.

3. Mild sore throat.

4. Watery eyes.

5. Decreased appetite, particularly in infants.

B. **Signs**

1. Erythematous, edematous nasal mucosa, with clear, thin nasal discharge initially. The discharge may become mucoid or purulent as the illness resolves.

2. Mildly erythematous pharynx.

3. Mild conjunctivitis.

4. Sometimes, fever. It is usually of low grade, but may be elevated in infants.

5. Erythematous tympanic membranes in infants.

IV. **Laboratory studies**

A. Usually, none.

B. Nasal culture for group A beta-hemolytic streptococci if nasal discharge persists for more than 2 weeks in an infant under 2 years of age and is associated with anorexia, fever, cervical lymphadenopathy, or, especially, excoriation and crusting around the nostrils.

V. **Differential diagnosis**

A. Allergic rhinitis.

B. Foreign body, particularly if nasal discharge is unilateral and malodorous, purulent, or bloody.

VI. **Treatment**

A. **Increased oral fluid intake.**

B. **Aspiration of nasal secretions** with rubber suction bulb in infants, particularly before feedings.

C. **Antipyretics and analgesics**

1. **Children under 12 years of age** Acetaminophen (Tylenol) or aspirin as needed for high fever (see Tables 5-9 and 5-10).

2. **Adults and children over 12 years of age**

a. Aspirin (325 mg per tablet), 1 or 2 tablets as often as every 4 hours

   or

b. Acetaminophen (325 mg per tablet), 1 or 2 tablets as often as every 6 hours.

Table 5-9   Oral Pediatric Dosage of Acetaminophen (Tylenol

| Age | Dose | | Frequency |
	Drops	Elixir	
3 months–1 year	0.6 ml	*or* 2.5 ml	As often a every 6 hours
1–3 years	0.6–1.2 ml	*or* 2.5–5 ml	
3–6 years	1.2 ml	*or* 5.0 ml	
Over 6 years	. . .	10.0 ml	

Table 5-10   Oral Pediatric Dosage of Aspirin

Body Weight	No. of 81-mg (1¼ grain) Tablets	Frequency
7–11 kg (14–24 lb)	1	As often a every 4 hours
11–16 kg (24–35 lb)	2	
16–23 kg (35–50 lb)	3	
Over 23 kg (over 50 lb)	4	

D. Medications for nasal stuffiness or discharge

1. **Children under 12 years of age**   Note   The nasal stuffiness and discharge of the common cold are self-limited and most patients do not need medication. When symptoms are causing distress or poor feeding or the child has had recurrent otitis media, medication *may* be helpful:

   a. Oral decongestant (see Table 5-5)

      or

   b. Oral antihistaminic-decongestant combination (see Table 5-6)

2. **Adults and children over 12 years of age**

   a. Oral decongestant: Pseudoephedrine (Sudafed) tablets (60 m per tablet), 1 tablet 3 or 4 times a day.

      or

   b. Oral antihistaminic-decongestant combination

      (1)   Brompheniramine-phenylephrine-phenylpropanolamine extended action tablets (Dimetapp Extentabs), 1 tablet twice a day

         or

      (2)   Triprolidine HCl and pseudoephedrine HCl (Actifed) tablets, 1 tablet 3 times a day.

and/or

c. Local decongestant: 0.1% xylometazoline (Otrivin) nasal spray, one spray followed in 5–10 minutes by a second spray; repeat sequence every 6 hours.

VII. Complications

A. Serous or purulent otitis media, particularly in infants and young children.

B. Sinusitis.

C. Lower respiratory tract infection.

VIII. Consultation – referral Only if indicated for a complication.

IX. Follow-up As needed.

6

Disorders of the Lower Respiratory System

ACUTE LARYNGOTRACHEOBRONCHITIS (VIRAL CROUP)
(Pediatric)

I. Definition Inflammation of the larynx often extending to the sub-glottis, trachea, and bronchi characterized by hoarseness, barking cough, and inspiratory stridor, usually occurring between ages 6 months and 5 years.

II. Etiology Myxoviruses (paramyxovirus types 1, 2, and 3 and influenza virus types A and B).

II. Clinical features

   A. Symptoms

      1. Barking cough.

      2. Inspiratory stridor.

      3. Hoarseness.

      4. Labored breathing.

      5. Nocturnal attacks or worsening of the disorder.

      6. Common cold symptoms usually preceding onset.

   B. Signs

      1. Inspiratory stridor.

      2. Barking cough.

      3. Hoarseness.

      4. Labored breathing with respiratory distress.

      5. Low-grade or absent fever.

V. Diagnostic studies Chest and lateral neck x-ray films only after consultation, but usually these are not needed.

V. Differential diagnosis

   A. Acute epiglottitis, suggested by the following:

      1. Fever over 101° F rectally.

2. Sudden onset, with rapid progression.

3. Severe respiratory distress.

4. Toxicity, agitation, or prostration.

5. Drooling with sore throat or difficulty swallowing, or both.

Note Do *not* attempt to look at the epiglottis or upset the patient. This can lead to complete obstruction.

B. Congenital laryngeal stridor in infant.

C. Aspirated foreign body.

D. Diphtheria.

VI. **Treatment**

A. Change environmental air to increase humidity:

1. Let patient breathe outside air when symptoms increase (usually at night).

2. Place patient in a steam-filled room, e.g., bathroom where hot water had been running.

B. Increase fluid intake.

VII. **Complications**

A. Airway obstruction.

B. Severe tracheobronchitis.

C. Pneumonia.

VIII. **Consultation — referral**

A. Signs of epiglottitis. *Refer immediately — this is an emergency.*

B. Respiratory distress.

IX. **Follow-up** Return visit if there is an increase in symptoms.

ACUTE TRACHEOBRONCHITIS (Pediatric)

I. **Definition** Acute inflammation of the respiratory epithelium of the trachea and bronchi without involvement of the alveoli or supporting lung tissue.

II. **Etiology**

A. A viral etiology is most common, particularly in young children.

Any of the viral respiratory pathogens may be responsible, but the myxoviruses (the paramyxoviruses and influenza virus types A and B) are most common.

B. *Mycoplasma pneumoniae* is a common cause in school-age children and adolescents.

III. Clinical features

A. Symptoms

1. Cough (persistent, dry, and worse at night).

2. Sometimes, mild tachypnea.

3. Restlessness and irritability associated with cough.

4. Sometimes, preceding or accompanying symptoms of upper respiratory tract infection.

5. Sometimes, systemic symptoms, including myalgia, headache, anorexia, and lethargy, particularly with influenza viruses.

B. Signs

1. Rhonchi.

2. High-pitched inspiratory or expiratory wheezing that improves with coughing.

3. Fever — usually absent or of low grade; sometimes high, particularly with influenza viruses.

4. Often, preceding or accompanying signs of upper respiratory tract infection.

IV. Diagnostic studies Chest x-ray only after consultation. Usually x-ray not needed.

V. Differential diagnosis

A. Uncomplicated upper respiratory tract infection.

B. Pneumonia.

C. Bronchial asthma.

D. Viral croup (laryngotracheobronchitis).

E. Allergic basis for cough.

F. Aspirated irritants, particularly hydrocarbons.

G. Aspirated foreign body.

H. Tuberculosis and other chronic pulmonary diseases.

I. Congestive heart failure.

VI. Treatment

A. Increased oral fluid intake.

B. Adequate environmental humidity.

C. Soothing preparations such as lemon juice mixed with honey.

D. Do not use antibiotics, as most cases are of viral origin.

E. Tuberculin skin test

   1. If there has not been one in a year.

   2. If there is a question of exposure to tuberculosis.

   3. If symptoms persist.

F. Acetaminophen or aspirin for fever (see Tables 5-9 and 5-10 for dosage).

VII. Complications

A. Usually, none.

B. Rarely, bacterial pneumonia.

VIII. Consultation — referral

A. Respiratory distress.

B. More than two episodes in a year.

C. Symptoms lasting more than 3 weeks.

D. Suspicion of aspiration.

IX. Follow-up

A. Clinic visit if no improvement in 7 days.

B. Children with chronic cardiorespiratory disease should be seen again in 2—3 days.

C. Return visit if symptoms of respiratory distress develop.

ACUTE BRONCHITIS (Adult)

I. **Definition**   An inflammatory disease of the bronchi characterized by one or more of the following: hyperemia of the bronchial mucosa, increased production of mucus, an inflammatory exudate of mucus and white blood cells.

II. Etiology   Viruses are the most common cause.

III. Clinical features

   A. Symptoms

      1. Cough is almost always present.

      2. The amount and character of sputum produced is of particular importance. Viral bronchitis rarely causes greater than 1 tablespoon per day of sputum, which is mucopurulent. Bacterial bronchitis is associated with purulent sputum, often greater than 1 tablespoon per day.

      3. Chest pain generally is a substernal discomfort aggravated by coughing.

      4. There are no frank, shaking chills.

      5. Dyspnea and wheezing may be present.

   B. Signs

      1. Temperature is usually less than $101°$ F.

      2. The chest is clear to percussion.

      3. Rhonchi or wheezing, or both, are present.

      4. Scattered rales may be present.

IV. Laboratory and other studies

   A. Sputum

      1. Sputum is initially clear in viral or mycoplasmal bronchitis, but purulent in bacterial bronchitis.

      2. Gram's stain and culture of sputum usually is not necessary unless sputum is purulent or pneumonia is suspected.

   B. A chest film may be taken if the clinical assessment is equivocal. Generally x-ray is not necessary, however.

   C. Blood count

      1. A white blood cell count is indicated only if the clinical picture is confusing. Consult with physician.

2. The white blood cell count usually is normal in viral or myco-plasmal disease; the count is rarely elevated, even in bacterial bronchitis.

V. **Differential diagnosis**

   A. Severe bronchopneumonia.

   B. Tuberculosis and other chronic pulmonary diseases.

   C. Bronchial asthma.

   D. Congestive heart failure.

VI. **Treatment**

   A. Bronchitis with production of less than 2 tablespoons of mucoid o mucopurulent sputum per day

      1. Rest.

      2. Aspirin for discomfort.

      3. Vaporizer or humidifier for moisture.

      4. Expectorant: Cough suppressants in the form of codeine or dextromethorphan hydrobromide should be used sparingly. Glyceryl guaiacolate may be used, although there is debate as to the efficacy of any expectorant.

   B. Bronchitis with production of greater than 2 tablespoons of purule sputum per day (usually associated with systemic symptoms)

      1. Rest.

      2. Aspirin for discomfort.

      3. Expectorant (see **VI.A.4**).

      4. Vaporizer or humidifier for moisture; this is of most value in winter.

      5. Antibiotic

         a. Ampicillin, 500 mg orally every 6 hours
            or
         b. Tetracycline, 250 mg orally every 6 hours.

      6. Bronchodilator (if significant wheezing is present): Aminophyl 200 mg 4 times a day.

      7. Removal of bronchial irritants.

VII. **Complications**   Generally none in simple bronchitis in adults.

III. **Consultation – referral**

    A. Significant respiratory distress.

    B. Failure to improve in 72 hours.

    C. Elderly patients, particularly those with chronic cardiovascular or pulmonary diseases, who have evidence of worsening cardiovascular status.

IX. **Follow-up**   Return visit if no improvement occurs in 72 hours, fever increases, or pleuritic pain develops.

INFLUENZA (Adult)

  I. **Definition**   An acute contagious viral illness often occurring in epidemics and characterized by fever, malaise, myalgia, and respiratory symptoms.

 II. **Etiology**   One or another of three myxoviruses having similar properties and categorized as influenza virus types A, B, and C. Influenza A viruses have shown an unusual ability to mutate, resulting in new antigenic strains that frequently produce worldwide epidemics.

III. **Clinical features**

    A. **Symptoms**

        1. Headache.

        2. Malaise, lassitude, and occasionally prostration.

        3. Myalgia.

        4. Nonproductive cough.

    B. **Signs**

        1. Fever, often $102°-103°$ F.

        2. Rhonchi and, occasionally, scattered rales.

IV. **Laboratory studies**   Generally, none.

 V. **Differential diagnosis**

    A. Other viral illnesses.

    B. Bacterial pneumonia.

    C. Other acute infectious illnesses.

VI. **Treatment**

A. Aspirin, 2 tablets orally every 4–6 hours for fever and myalgia.

B. Increased fluid intake.

C. Mild cough suppressant, such as Robitussin-DM (glycerol guaiacola
and dextromethorphan hydrobromide), 2 teaspoons orally every
4–6 hours as needed for cough.

VII. Complications

A. Influenzal pneumonia.

B. Secondary bacterial pneumonia.

C. Rarely, encephalitis and myocarditis.

VIII. Consultation – referral

A. Severely ill patients, particularly the elderly.

B. Respiratory distress or widespread rales or rhonchi on physical
examination, or both of these.

C. Pregnant patients.

IX. Follow-up   As needed.

BRONCHIAL ASTHMA (Pediatric)

I. Definition   A reversible obstructive airway disease characterized clinic
by intermittent episodes of cough, dyspnea, and prolonged expiration
with wheezing.

II. Etiology   Bronchial asthma may be of single, multiple, or unknown
cause. The precipitating factor may not necessarily be the same in eac
episode. Each attack may be associated with one or a combination of
the factors listed below:

A. Allergy – inhalant (dust, mold, pollen) or food (especially in infan

B. Acute or chronic infection – viral, bacterial, fungal.

C. Weather changes – rising pressure and decreasing temperature,
changes in humidity and wind velocity.

D. Extreme exertion.

E. Nonspecific irritants – chemical fumes, air pollution, tobacco smok

F. Psychogenic factors.

III. **Clinical features**   The amount of airway obstruction determines the severity of symptoms and signs.

   A. **Symptoms**

      1. Cough.

      2. Dyspnea or chest tightness, anxiety, apprehension.

      3. Wheezing.

      4. Occasionally, vomiting following paroxysmal coughing.

      5. Abdominal pain associated with coughing or respiratory distress.

      6. Family history of allergic disease.

   B. **Signs**

      1. Prolonged expiration with expiratory and occasionally inspiratory wheezes.

      2. Hyperresonant percussion note.

      3. Tachypnea.

      4. Sometimes, inspiratory and expiratory rhonchi or rales, or both.

      5. Intercostal retractions.

      6. Use of accessory muscles of respiration, e.g., sternomastoids and diaphragm.

      7. Increased anteroposterior diameter of chest.

      8. Cyanosis in severe attack.

      9. Sometimes, with respiratory failure and decreased effort, less labored respirations, less audible wheezes, and death.

      10. Fever, if infection is present.

      11. Evidence of upper respiratory tract infection.

      12. Sometimes, evidence of other allergic diseases, e.g., allergic rhinitis and atopic dermatitis.

IV. **Diagnostic studies**   Chest x-ray only after consultation. X-ray is not needed in most cases.

V. **Differential diagnosis**

   A. Acute bronchiolitis of infancy.

   B. Aspirated foreign body (e.g., peanut), especially in young children with unilateral findings, although asthma can be associated with differences in findings in the two lung fields.

C. Bronchospasm associated with pneumonia.

D. Parasitic infestation: ascariasis, visceral larva migrans.

VI. Treatment

A. Moderate to severe acute attack

1. Administer aqueous epinephrine, 1:1000, for bronchodilatation

    a. Inject 0.01 ml per kg (0.005 ml per lb), with a maximum dose of 0.3 ml, subcutaneously into the upper arm.

    b. If wheezes are still present after 20 minutes, repeat the dose epinephrine. Do not delay the repeat dose beyond 20 minutes if no side-effects are present.

    c. Delay the second dose if side-effects (tremor, tachycardia, anxiety, sweating) develop.

    d. Document the effect of each dose by recording pulse, respirations, symptoms, auscultatory findings, and time of injection

2. Try to calm and reassure the patient, as anxiety can increase bronchospasm.

3. Administer oxygen for cyanosis.

4. Encourage increased oral fluid intake.

5. If the patient is not significantly relieved by the preceding regimen consult the physician.

6. If the patient is significantly relieved and ready for discharge from the clinic, proceed with the following:

    a. Aqueous epinephrine suspension, 1:200, (Sus-Phrine) for sustained (8–10 hours) bronchodilatation. Inject 0.005 ml per (0.0025 ml per lb) subcutaneously after shaking the vial; maximum dose is 0.15 ml.

    b. Maintenance therapy (see **B**).

B. Mild attack and home maintenance therapy

1. Use theophylline preparation for bronchodilatation:

    a. For children less than 40 kg, use oral theophylline preparation (see Table 6-1).

b. For children over 40 kg (over 88 lb), give aminophylline tablets (100 mg per tablet) in a dosage of 200 mg (2 tablets) every 6 hours. Continue for 2 weeks *after* all symptoms and signs have disappeared.

2. Encourage intake of large amounts of clear liquids.

3. Manage or counsel to avoid the precipitating factors that apply to the patient. Emotional stress and physical exertion should be avoided during an asthmatic attack, regardless of the underlying cause.

4. Suggest that the patient and his family keep a diary when attacks occur to discover precipitating factors.

II. Complications of acute attack

A. Hypoxia.

B. Atelectasis.

C. Pneumonia.

D. Dehydration.

E. Pneumothorax or pneumomediastinum, or both.

F. Respiratory failure.

G. Death.

III. Consultation — referral

A. Failure of an acute attack to respond to treatment.

B. Persistent wheezing at follow-up visit despite maintenance therapy.

Table 6-1 Oral Dosage of Theophylline Preparations for Children less than 40 Kg (88 lb) for Bronchodilatation

Drug Type	Body Weight	Dose	Frequency
Theophylline elixir (Elixophyllin)	15−20 kg (33−44 lb)	15 ml	Every 6 hours. Continue for 2 weeks after all symptoms and signs have disappeared.
	20−27 kg (44−60 lb)	20 ml	
	27−34 kg (60−75 lb)	25 ml	
	34−40 kg (75−88 lb)	30 ml	
Oxtriphylline elixir (Choledyl)	15−20 kg (33−44 lb)	6 ml	
	20−27 kg (44−60 lb)	8 ml	
	27−34 kg (60−75 lb)	10 ml	
	34−40 kg (75−88 lb)	12 ml	

    C. Repeated attacks (more than two per year).

 IX. Follow-up Return visit in 10–14 days; sooner if there is no improve

BRONCHIAL ASTHMA
(Acute Attack in a Known Adult Asthmatic)

 I. Definition A reversible clinical syndrome characterized by episodes c wheezing and dyspnea separated by intervals of normal breathing.

 II. Etiology An acute attack of bronchial asthma may be of a single, multiple, or unknown cause. Each attack may be associated with one a combination of the factors listed below. The precipitating factor m; not necessarily be the same in each episode.

    A. Allergy – inhalant, food.

    B. Acute or chronic infection – viral, bacterial, tuberculous, fungal.

    C. Environmental physical factors – humidity, temperature, dust, fumes, odors.

    D. Exertion.

    E. Psychogenic factors.

III. Clinical features

    A. Symptoms

       1. History of frequent episodes of eczema or atopic dermatitis.

       2. Cough.

       3. Dyspnea.

       4. Wheezing.

    B. Signs

       1. Prolonged expiration with expiratory and occasionally inspiratc wheezes.

       2. Tachypnea.

       3. Use of accessory muscles of respiration, e.g., sternomastoids an scalenus.

       4. Intercostal retractions.

   5. Perspiration.

   6. Cyanosis, with severe asthma.

   7. Hyperresonant percussion note.

   8. Presence of the following, depending on etiology:

      a. Fever.

      b. Rhinorrhea.

      c. Evidence of upper respiratory tract infection or allergy.

IV. **Laboratory and other studies** In general no laboratory studies are indicated. If infection is suspected, the following should be initiated and a consultation obtained.

   A. Chest x-ray, to demonstrate:

      1. Hyperinflation.

      2. Evidence of pulmonary infection.

      3. Cardiac enlargement and evidence of heart failure if underlying heart disease is severe.

   B. White blood cell count and differential count

      1. Eosinophils may be elevated if allergic reaction is an important component of the asthma.

      2. If the white blood cell count is very high, acute infection should be suspected.

   C. Microscopic examination of sputum

      1. Presence of polyps and bacteria should raise suspicion of acute infection.

      2. Wright's stain of sputum will show large numbers of eosinophils if allergic reaction is an important component of the asthma.

   D. Culture of sputum

      1. *Hemophilus influenzae* and pneumococcus are important pathogens.

      2. "Normal" flora (*Neisseria* and alpha-hemolytic streptococci) may be the cause of an acute attack.

V. **Differential diagnosis**

A. Acute bronchitis: Sometimes this is hard to differentiate from acute asthma; in general, the history of previous attacks or previous chronic obstructive pulmonary disease (COPD) coupled with the mode of onset may indicate asthma.

B. Aspirated foreign body.

C. Pneumonia.

D. Allergic reaction to drug, inhalant, or food (anaphylaxis), especially the syndrome of chronic sinusitis, nasal polyps, and asthma that is associated with aspirin ingestion.

E. Congestive heart failure (sometimes called *cardiac asthma*) may mimic allergic asthma closely.

F. Pulmonary emboli.

VI. **Treatment**   The following regimen is intended for young to middle-aged patients with known asthma and no heart disease. **Warning** Asthma may deteriorate into status asthmaticus in hours.

A. Give water orally during therapy.

B. Do not use sedatives without consulting physician.

C. Initially give 0.2–0.3 ml of 1:1000 aqueous epinephrine subcutaneously; reassess in 15–20 minutes and then repeat the dose if the attack persists. Up to three injections may be given, with assessment between each injection.

D. If epinephrine therapy (C) is successful:

1. Inject 0.3 ml of Sus-Phrine subcutaneously.

2. Begin maintenance therapy.

    a. Aminophylline tablets: 200 mg 4 times a day. (If nocturnal dyspnea is a problem, use an aminophylline suppository [250–500 mg] at bedtime.)

    or

    b. Theophylline

    (1)   Capsules: 200 mg 4 times a day

    or

    (2)   Elixir: 2 tablespoons 4 times a day.

3. Use antibiotics if infection is significant component of the asthma

        a. Tetracycline, 250 mg orally 4 times a day

        or

        b. Ampicillin, 500 mg orally 4 times a day (if patient is not allergic to penicillin).

    4. Expectorant, such as glyceryl guaiacolate, is commonly used but of undocumented value.

    5. Continue inhalants if patient has been on them, e.g., isoproterenol (Isuprel).

  E. If A–D are not successful, consult physician.

VII. Complications

  A. Severe hypoxia.

  B. Dehydration.

  C. Atelectasis.

  D. Pneumonia.

  E. Pneumothorax or pneumomediastinum, or both.

  F. Respiratory failure.

VIII. Consultation – referral

  A. All new cases, whether the patient's first attack or the first time the patient has been seen.

  B. All asthmatics over 60 years of age.

  C. All asthmatics with history of heart disease.

  D. All patients known to have COPD, if any significant respiratory distress is present.

  E. Patients in whom therapy fails.

  F. Extreme shortness of breath.

IX. Follow-up
Patients should be followed regularly every 1 to 3 months and seen promptly whenever necessary for acute attacks and/or symptoms or signs of infection.

CHRONIC OBSTRUCTIVE PULMONARY DISEASE (Adult)

I. **Definition** A complex syndrome of decreased pulmonary function made up of three components in various combinations: emphysema characterized by irreversible destruction of the distal airspace, bronchitis characterized by excessive mucus production and inflammation of the bronchi resulting in sputum production, and asthma. Any of the three may predominate.

II. **Etiology** Unknown. Most cases are strongly associated with a history of smoking.

III. **Clinical features**

A. **Symptoms**

1. Shortness of breath, first noticeable with exertion.

2. Chronic cough and sputum production, frequently in the morning.

3. Often, episodes of wheezing.

B. **Signs**

1. Early, no clinical signs.

2. Tachypnea, somewhat labored, with loud breathing. As the disease progresses, there are increasing signs of hyperinflation and obstruction, depending on the composition of the disease.

3. Increased anteroposterior diameter of the chest.

4. Hyperresonant percussion note.

5. Frequently, rhonchi.

6. Wheezing.

7. Distant heart sounds.

8. Decreased lateral movement of the thorax with increase in upward vector of the sternum.

9. Decreased diaphragmatic movement.

10. Use of the accessory muscles of respiration.

11. Sometimes in severe disease, paradoxical inward movement of the lower costal margins.

IV. **Diagnostic studies**

A. Chest x-ray.

B. Spirometry: FEV and MMFR.

    C. Sputum culture (occasionally helpful).

    D. Electrocardiogram.

V. Differential diagnosis

    A. Allergic asthma.

    B. Acute bronchitis.

    C. Congestive heart failure.

VI. Treatment

    A. Prevention Yearly immunization with influenza vaccine.

    B. Stable chronic disease

      1. **Avoidance of pulmonary irritants,** especially cigarettes.

      2. **Bronchodilator** Almost all patients with chronic obstructive pulmonary disease have some element of bronchospasm. Use aminophylline, 200 mg orally 4 times a day indefinitely.

      3. **Expectorants** There is doubt as to whether these do any more good than moisturizing with steam.

        a. Glyceryl guaiacolate, 2 teaspoons by mouth every 4–6 hours.

        b. Saturated solution of potassium iodide, 15 drops in a glass of water 3 times a day.

        c. Vaporizer.

      4. **Avoidance of sedatives.**

      5. A routine of **postural drainage** 3 or 4 times a day

        a. Drink a hot cup of coffee or tea.

        b. Use a vaporizer for 5–10 minutes.

        c. Take an expectorant.

        d. Proceed with postural drainage in four positions, staying in each position for 5 minutes:

          (1) Supine.

          (2) Right side down.

          (3) Left side down.

          (4) Prone with head down at a 30-degree angle.

C. Acute attack (manifested by increased symptoms, fever, and change in color and quantity of sputum)

1. **Consult physician.**

2. **General therapy** as for chronic disease (see **B**).

3. **Hydration and humidification** (extremely important).

4. **Antibiotics**

   a. Tetracycline, 250 mg orally every 6 hours

   or

   b. Ampicillin, 500 mg orally every 6 hours.

5. **Discretionary chest x-ray.** Unsuspected pneumonia is common.

VII. Complications

A. Pneumonia.

B. Respiratory failure.

C. Cor pulmonale.

VIII. Consultation — referral

A. All new cases of suspected COPD.

B. Pneumonia.

C. Coexisting acute or chronic bronchitis if the patient has any significant change in respiratory function or a temperature greater than 101° F.

D. Failure to improve within 48 hours.

E. Suspected respiratory failure, manifested by severe dyspnea or any confusion or clouding of consciousness, or both.

IX. Follow-up

A. **Acute attack**   Telephone call if there is no improvement in 3 days or immediately if condition worsens.

B. **Stable chronic disease**

1. In 3 months for review.

2. Repeat spirometry every year.

3. Emphasize to the patient the importance of consulting the FNP or physician promptly. Development of symptoms or signs of respiratory infection or increased shortness of breath, or both.

ACUTE BRONCHIOLITIS (Pediatric)

I. **Definition**   A generalized inflammation of the bronchioles, characterized by signs of expiratory obstruction, occurring usually as an epidemic
disease in winter and early spring in children under 3 years.

II. **Etiology**

   A. Epidemic forms are usually caused by respiratory syncytial virus.

   B. Sporadic cases are usually viral in origin, but bacteria, allergy, and
   Mycoplasma pneumoniae may be responsible.

III. **Clinical features**

   A. **Symptoms**

      1. Onset as an upper respiratory tract infection.

      2. Paroxysmal coughing.

      3. Expiratory wheezing.

      4. Dyspnea.

      5. Difficulty sleeping and feeding.

   B. **Signs**

      1. Rapid respirations.

      2. Symmetric expiratory wheezing or grunting, or both.

      3. Air-trapping causing liver to be pushed down, hyperresonant
      percussion note, and prolonged expiratory phase.

      4. Increased heart rate.

      5. Sometimes, fever (usually of low grade).

      6. Sometimes, rales.

IV. **Diagnostic studies**   Chest x-ray only after consultation.   Usually x-ray
is not needed.

V. **Differential diagnosis**

   A. Pneumonia.

   B. Asthmatic bronchitis.

   C. Tracheobronchitis.

   D. Pertussis.

      E. Aspirated foreign body, especially with unilateral signs.

VI. Treatment

      A. Cool, moist air from a vaporizer, if available.

      B. Increased fluid intake.

      C. Therapeutic trial of epinephrine after physician consultation when asthmatic bronchitis is suspected (recurrent episodes, older infant, strong allergic family history).

VII. Complications

      A. Hypoxia.

      B. Progressive exhaustion followed by respiratory failure.

      C. Dehydration from loss of water through lungs combined with poor intake (usually in infant under 4 months of age).

      D. Superimposed bacterial infection.

VIII. Consultation – referral

      A. Respiratory distress.

      B. Children under 3 months of age.

      C. More than two episodes. Refer for evaluation of possible underlying causes.

IX. Follow-up Return visit if there is no improvement in 48 hours.

PNEUMONIA (Pediatric)

I. Definition Inflammation of the lung involving the alveoli or interstitial tissues, or both.

II. Etiology

      A. A viral etiology is most common, particularly in preschool children. Respiratory syncytial virus and paramyxovirus type 3 are particularly common causes in children under 3 years of age.

      B. *Mycoplasma pneumoniae* probably accounts for at least half of the cases of pneumonia seen in school-age children, adolescents, and young adults. It is usually characterized by insidious onset and mild disease.

      C. Bacterial pneumonia is less common than viral pneumonia and is usually due to pneumococcus, *Hemophilus influenzae,* or, rarely,

Staphylococcus aureus. Marked toxicity and consolidation or pleural fluid are usually present.

III. **Clinical features**

A. **Symptoms**

1. Upper respiratory tract infection that precedes or accompanies the pneumonia.

2. Cough.

3. Fever.

4. Rapid or labored breathing, or both.

5. Lethargy.

6. Anorexia.

7. Abdominal pain and distention.

8. Vomiting.

B. **Signs**

1. Rapid breathing.

2. Labored breathing

a. Grunting on expiration.

b. Flaring of nostrils.

c. Intercostal and subcostal retractions.

3. Fine, crackling rales.

4. Evidence of consolidation or pleural effusion, or both

a. Decreased breath sounds.

b. Dullness to percussion.

5. Sometimes, marked fever, lethargy, and anorexia.

IV. **Diagnostic studies** Chest x-ray only after consultation. X-ray is not needed in mild cases.

V. **Differential diagnosis**

A. Bronchiolitis and tracheobronchitis.

B. Aspirated foreign body.

C. Tuberculosis.

VI. Treatment

A. Increased fluid intake.

B. Rest, as needed.

C. Acetaminophen or aspirin for fever (see Tables 5-9 and 5-10 for dosage).

D. Antibiotics for bacterial or mycoplasmal disease, after consultation

VII. Complications

A. Empyema.

B. Atelectasis.

C. Bronchiectasis.

D. Pneumothorax.

E. Dehydration.

VIII. Consultation — referral

A. All cases of pneumonia.

B. Failure to improve in 48 hours.

C. Failure to resolve in 3 weeks.

IX. Follow-up

A. Telephone call, home visit, or clinic visit every day until patient is afebrile and has no respiratory distress.

B. Return visit in 3 weeks.

C. Repeat chest x-ray for severe disease or persisting symptoms and signs. Consult physician for review of initial x-ray film for decision concerning the necessity and timing of follow-up films.

7

Disorders of the Cardiovascular System

ANGINA PECTORIS (Adult)

I. **Definition** Pain, usually in the substernal region of the chest but occasionally in the epigastrium, or neck, per **III.A.1**, or back, that is caused by an imbalance between the work required for the myocardium and the oxygen supply to the myocardium.

II. **Etiology** Usually, atherosclerosis of the coronary arteries.

III. **Clinical features**

A. **Symptoms** Diagnosis is based primarily on the nature of the pain.

1. **Location** Pain is usually located in the substernal region of the chest but occasionally is present in the epigastrium, neck, back, or arms.

2. **Onset** Pain occurs with an increase in the work load on the heart and is relieved by a decrease in the work load. Classically, this is demonstrated by pain occurring with work and relieved by rest (usually within 3—5 minutes).

3. **Description** The pain is usually described as squeezing or pressure-like, sometimes as expanding, and seldom as sticking, sharp, or burning.

4. **Radiating pain** Pain often radiates to the neck, shoulder, or arms (the left arm more often than the right).

5. **Accompanying symptoms** Sometimes there is slight shortness of breath, mild diaphoresis, or slight nausea, or a combination of these. The pain is not pleuritic.

B. **Signs** There are no signs in uncomplicated angina. Nonetheless, one should carefully examine the heart and lungs for signs of congestive heart failure, valvular heart disease, etc.

IV. **Diagnostic studies** Electrocardiogram may show no abnormality, particularly during attack of pain. It may, however, be completely normal.

V. **Differential diagnosis**

A. Acute myocardial infarction.

     B. Preinfarctional angina.

     C. Musculoskeletal pain (e.g., costochondritis).

     D. Esophagitis, esophageal spasm, and other gastrointestinal causes of chest pain.

     E. Pleurisy and other pulmonary causes of chest pain.

     F. Psychosomatic chest pain.

     G. Malingering.

     H. Cervical spine root compression.

VI. Treatment   Angina pectoris can be divided into two broad categories, *stable angina* and *unstable angina,* which are treated differently:

     A. Stable angina is previously diagnosed angina that recurs with approximately the same amount of exertion and the same frequency and intensity of pain and is relieved after approximately the same period of rest (less than 15 minutes).

       1. General measures

         a. Reduction of the work load on the heart

           (1) Reduction of exertion performed by the patient until attacks are infrequent or absent.

           (2) Reduction of work load by control of other diseases that tend to increase the work load

              (a) Control of hypertension (see Uncomplicated Essential Hypertension [Adult]).

              (b) Correction of anemia.

              (c) Treatment of anxiety.

         b. Improvement of cardiac performance without changing work load

           (1) Treatment leading to compensation of congestive heart failure (see Congestive Heart Failure [Adult], **VI**).

           (2) Correction of valvular heart disease.

       2. Specific therapy

         a. Nitroglycerine, one 0.4–0.6-mg tablet sublingually every 3–5 minutes until pain is relieved or headache results; not to exceed a total of 3 tablets.

  b. Long-acting nitrites. Consult physician.

 B. Unstable angina consists of angina de novo (the first attack or attacks of angina) or a worsening of previously stable angina characterized by more severe or persistent pain, pain on less exertion, or pain at rest. These patients should be *referred* and hospitalization considered.

VII. Complications

 A. Myocardial infarction.

 B. Congestive heart failure.

 C. Cardiac neurosis.

III. Consultation – referral

 A. Unstable angina, including angina de novo.

 B. Development of congestive heart failure.

 C. Elevated serum cholesterol and triglyceride levels.

 D. Angina requiring more than 3 nitroglycerin tablets for relief.

 E. Angina persisting more than 20 minutes.

IX. Follow-up and maintenance of stable angina

 A. Frequency of assessment This can vary considerably, depending on the severity of the disease and the presence or absence of other conditions, such as hypertension, congestive heart failure, etc. For angina uncomplicated by other problems, a visit every 2–4 months should be adequate. *Any time angina becomes unstable (see* **VI.B***), the patient should seek care.*

 B. Content of assessment

  1. Subjective evaluation

   a. Stability of angina.

   b. Symptoms of congestive heart failure.

   c. Response to nitroglycerine, and complications such as headache.

  2. Objective evaluation

   a. Assessment of heart and lungs, particularly for signs of congestive heart failure.

   b. ECG every year.

CONGESTIVE HEART FAILURE (Adult)

I. **Definition**   A complicated state of altered cardiac function in which there is inadequate cardiac output to meet the demand for oxygen of metabolizing tissues leading to an excessive retention of salt and water.

II. **Etiology**   Any process that damages the heart. In the United States, the most common causes are arteriosclerotic heart disease and hypertensive heart disease.

III. **Clinical features**

A. **Symptoms**

1. Dyspnea on exertion.

2. Orthopnea.

3. Paroxysmal nocturnal dyspnea.

4. Ankle swelling.

5. Nocturia: In diabetes and congestive heart failure, patients pass large volumes of urine. In benign prostatic hypertrophy there is frequent, difficult voiding of small amounts of urine.

B. **Signs**

1. Tachycardia.

2. Weight gain, reflecting fluid retention.

3. Neck vein distention.

4. Rales, particularly over the lower chest.

5. Gallop rhythm.

6. Bilateral dependent edema.

7. Hepatomegaly with severe, usually chronic heart failure.

8. Rarely, ascites.

IV. **Laboratory and diagnostic studies**

A. Chest x-ray may be helpful in diagnosing questionable cases or better assessing the magnitude of the problem.

B. An electrocardiogram may be helpful in determining the etiology; it is seldom helpful in establishing a diagnosis of failure or monitoring response to therapy.

C. Serum electrolyte and creatinine levels are useful as a baseline and should be measured before treatment is instituted.

V. Differential diagnosis

A. Other causes of dyspnea, such as chronic lung disease and asthma.

B. Other causes of edema, such as renal disease, liver disease, and local venous problems.

C. Recurrent pulmonary emboli.

D. Other causes of wheezes, such as asthma.

VI. Treatment
The general goal of therapy is to rid the body of excess salt and water by a combination of measures designed to **improve cardiac function** and to **increase renal excretion** of salt and water. The physician should be consulted before any treatment is begun.

A. Initial therapy

1. **Low-sodium diet** Generally, few patients can restrict their sodium intake below 85 mEq per day without major alterations in their style of living and eating. Usually, however, restriction to this level is adequate. In refractory cases further restriction should be attempted.

2. Measures designed to **improve myocardial function**

   a. Reduction of systemic blood pressure to normal levels if it is elevated. Consult physician for regimen.

   b. Correction of anemia, if present.

   c. Use of digitalis preparations, such as digoxin. Consult physician for initial dosage regimen and establishment of maintenance therapy (see **IX.C.1**).

3. Measures to **increase renal excretion** of sodium and water

   a. **Oral diuretics** if the patient is not acutely ill.

      (1) Hydrochlorothiazide, 25–50 mg every day. The dosage may be increased to 100 mg every day.

      (2) Chlorthalidone, 50–100 mg every day.

   b. **Intramuscular diuretics,** e.g., furosemide, 20–40 mg IM. These should not be used without physician consultation.

B. Maintenance therapy (see **IX.A**).

VII. Complications

A. Worsening CHF.

B. Arrhythmias.

C. Hepatomegaly, ascites, profound edema.

D. Pulmonary embolism.

E. Digitalis toxicity (see **IX.C.1**).

F. Side-effects of diuretics

1. Hypokalemia.

2. Hyperglycemia.

3. Hyperuricemia.

4. Increased blood urea nitrogen (prerenal azotemia).

5. Orthostatic hypotension.

G. Pulmonary infection.

VIII. Consultation – referral

A. All new patients should initially have a physician consultation.

B. All patients should be followed by FNP with close physician consultation until their condition is stable on the maintenance regimen. The FNP may then follow and alter the regimen as needed on the basis of the follow-up or maintenance guidelines (**IX**), but should consult frequently.

C. Worsening CHF.

D. Arrhythmia.

IX. Follow-up and maintenance

A. Frequency of assessment

1. Initial follow-up in 24 hours to determine if regimen has improved dynamics.

2. Then every 1–2 weeks until patient is symptom-free and dry weight is achieved.

3. Then every month for 3 months.

4. Then every 6–8 weeks indefinitely.

B. Content of assessment (related to basic diseases)

    1. Subjective symptoms

        a. Dyspnea on exertion.

        b. Orthopnea.

        c. Paroxysmal nocturnal dyspnea.

    2. Objective evaluation

        a. Neck veins – look for distention.

        b. Chest examination – listen for rales.

        c. Cardiac examination – listen for gallop rhythm.

        d. Abdomen – determine liver size.

        e. Extremities – check for edema.

        f. Weight (change in body weight is one of the most sensitive measurements of fluid balance).

C. Treatment

    1. Digitalis (Dosage or drug should not be altered without physician consultation.)

        a. Drug and usual maintenance dosage

            (1) Digoxin, 0.125–0.375 mg orally every day.

            (2) Digitoxin, 0.1 mg orally every day.

        b. Assessment related to digitalis

            (1) Subjective symptoms (assess at each visit)

                (a) Nausea, vomiting, anorexia.

                (b) "Yellow vision."

                (c) Palpitations.

            (2) Objective symptoms

                (a) Bradycardia of 60 beats or less (assess at each visit).

                (b) Arrhythmias, commonly premature ventricular contractions (assess at each visit).

                (c) Serum electrolytes every 3–6 months.

    2. Thiazide diuretics (see Uncomplicated Essential Hypertension [Adult], **VI.A.2**).

UNCOMPLICATED ESSENTIAL HYPERTENSION (Adult)

I. **Definition**   Persistent elevation of the arterial blood pressure greater than 150/100 mm Hg (present on weekly determinations over a period of 3 weeks) without demonstrable cause and with no associated symptoms or signs of end-organ involvement.

II. **Etiology**   Unknown.

III. **Clinical features**

A. **Symptoms**

1. Frequently the patient is asymptomatic.

2. The patient may have headaches. Typically these are occipital headaches, more severe in the early morning just after the patient arises and becoming less severe or disappearing after he is ambulatory for several hours.

3. The patient may experience dizziness that is better termed *unsteadiness* — it is *not* true vertigo.

4. In uncomplicated hypertension, the following symptoms of target organ involvement are *not* present:

   a. Symptoms of angina pectoris.

   b. Symptoms of congestive heart failure.

   c. Symptoms of cerebral ischemia or a stroke syndrome.

   d. Severe headaches, nausea, and vomiting.

   e. Alterations in level of consciousness.

B. **Signs**

1. Elevation of arterial blood pressure greater than 150/100 mm Hg

2. Sometimes, narrowing, copper-wiring, or arteriovenous nicking of the arterioles of the optic fundi. Usually there are no hemorrhages or exudates, and there is no papilledema.

3. Chest clear to percussion and auscultation.

4. Heart: The heart is usually normal, although it may show minimal to moderate left ventricular hypertrophy. No gallop rhythm is present.

5. No bruit over abdomen or flank or in back.

6. No edema.

7. Intact neurological system.

8. No signs of Cushing's syndrome, hyperthyroidism, or pheochromo-cytoma.

IV. Laboratory and other studies

A. Before treatment

1. Blood urea nitrogen or creatinine.

2. Serum sodium, potassium, carbon dioxide, and chloride levels.

3. Blood sugar concentration (preferably 2 hours after eating, or after fasting).

4. Electrocardiogram.

5. Chest x-ray.

6. Urinalysis.

7. Hypertensive intravenous pyelography, measurement of vanillyl-mandelic acid level, and other studies; these are deferred until the patient has been seen by the physician, or after consultation with the physician.

B. After treatment   (See treatment guidelines, VI.C.)

V. Differential diagnosis

A. Headaches and dizziness of other origin.

B. Secondary hypertension

1. Systolic hypertension

   a. Arteriosclerotic vascular disease.

   b. Hyperthyroidism.

   c. Anxiety.

2. Diastolic hypertension

   a. Renal disease.

   b. Coarctation of aorta.

   c. Pheochromocytoma.

   d. Cushing's syndrome.

VI. Treatment   The goal of treatment is the achievement and maintenanc of a normal blood pressure (110/70–140/90 mm Hg) and the preventi of complications of either the disease or the treatment regimens.

A. Initial therapy   If the patient meets the criteria as outlined for uncomplicated benign essential hypertension:

1. **Salt-restricted diet**   Salt intake should approximate 85 mEq (2 gm) sodium daily, but may be altered as necessary, depending on patient's socioeconomic status, habits of living and eating, ability to comprehend, etc.

2. **Thiazide diuretic**

   a. Hydrochlorothiazide

      (1)   Initial dosage is 50 mg orally every day.

      (2)   Dosage may be increased in 2 weeks to 50 mg orally twice a day.

   or

   b. Chlorthalidone

      (1)   Initial dosage is 50 mg orally every day.

      (2)   Dosage may be increased in 2 weeks to 100 mg orally every day.

B. Intermediate therapy   If initial therapy is not effective in bringing the blood pressure to normal levels, begin a second level of therapy consisting of **reserpine*** **plus a diuretic:**

1. Administer 50 mg thiazide and 0.25 mg reserpine orally every day.

2. Double the dosage in 1 month if necessary.

C. Follow-up and maintenance

1. Frequency of assessment

*Reserpine is chosen as the drug to be started at this intermediate level for several reasc It has few side-effects, is inexpensive, and need be given only once daily. As thiazide diuretics need also be given only once daily, there are rational combination tablets of reserpine and thiazide that require only 1 tablet a day. Compliance may be better if only 1 tablet is necessary. It is recognized that other antihypertensives may be used at this level and some physicians may wish to substitute another drug. Also, recent eviden suggests that reserpine may be associated with breast cancer; this aspect of reserpine therapy must be watched in the future.

    a. Every 1–2 weeks until normal blood pressure is achieved.

    b. Then every month for 3 months.

    c. Then every 3–4 months indefinitely.

2. Contents of assessment (related to hypertension)

  a. Subjective symptoms

    (1) Headaches.

    (2) Dizziness.

    (3) Angina.

    (4) Congestive heart failure.

    (5) Cerebral ischemia or stroke syndrome.

    (6) Nausea, vomiting.

    (7) Alterations of level of consciousness.

  b. Objective evaluation

    (1) Blood pressure — measure supine and standing at each visit.

    (2) Appropriate examination related to symptoms.

    (3) Routine examination of heart, lungs, and nervous system every 6 months.

3. Assessment related to thiazide

  a. Subjective symptoms (review at each visit)

    (1) Hypokalemia — lethargy, muscle cramps.

    (2) Gout — acute joint pain.

    (3) Diabetes — polyuria, etc.

  b. Objective evaluation

    (1) Orthostatic hypotension — obtain supine and standing blood pressure at each visit.

    (2) Serum potassium level — measure initially, repeat after diuretic dose is established, and repeat every 6 months thereafter.

       (3)   Serum uric acid level check any time joint pain develops. Check at end of the first 3 months of therapy and then annually.

       (4)   Blood sugar level — check if polydipsia, polyuria, or polyphagia develops. Check routinely at end of the first 3 months of therapy and then annually, 2 hours after eating.

    4. Assessment related to reserpine

      a. Subjective symptoms

        (1)   Nasal stuffiness.

        (2)   Depression.

        (3)   Epigastric pain.

        (4)   Impotence.

      b. Objective symptoms

        (1)   Stool benzidine test every month for 3 months, then once every 6 months.

        (2)   Hematocrit reading every month for 3 months, then once every 6 months.

VII. Complications

A. Angina pectoris.

B. Congestive heart failure.

C. Transient cerebral ischemia or other stroke syndrome.

D. Secondary renal disease.

E. Complications of therapy.

VIII. Consultation — referral

A. Any patient with hypertension who has a blood pressure of 170/110 mm Hg or any patient exhibiting symptoms or signs of complications of hypertension.

B. Any patient not controlled on maximum dosage of thiazide or reserpine plus a thiazide.

C. Any patient who has complications related to his treatment regimen.

IX. Follow-up   See VI.C.

CHRONIC OCCLUSIVE ARTERIAL DISEASE OF THE EXTREMITIES
(Adult)

I. **Definition** A disease characterized by a chronic decrease in blood flow to one or more of the extremities due to partial or complete occlusion of one or more of the peripheral blood vessels.

II. **Etiology** Usually atherosclerosis. Congenital lesions, trauma, and other mechanisms may be causative. It is a common complication of diabetes.

III. **Clinical features**

    A. **Symptoms** Symptoms depend on the level of occlusion. Thus, the following symptoms may occur in the buttocks, thigh, calf, or arm:

        1. Intermittent claudication due to cramping pain in the muscles on exercise. Pain is relieved by rest.

        2. Occasional nocturnal cramps.

        3. Feeling of coldness in involved extremity.

    B. **Signs**

        1. Decreased pulses in the involved extremity.

        2. Coolness of the involved extremity to the touch.

        3. Loss of hair on the involved extremity.

        4. Shiny, atrophic skin on the involved extremity.

        5. Ischemic necrosis (gangrene) in advanced disease.

        6. Bruits may be heard over the involved vessel, particularly the femoral arteries and abdominal aorta.

IV. **Laboratory studies**

    A. Urine and blood sugar levels to screen for diabetes mellitus.

    B. Fasting serum cholesterol and triglyceride levels.

V. **Differential diagnosis**

    A. Raynaud's disease.

    B. Raynaud's phenomenon.

    C. Scleroderma.

    D. Problems of venous stasis (see Stasis Ulcer of the Lower Extremity [Adult]).

VI. Treatment

A. The patient should be instructed in methods of good skin care usin[g] lanolin, lamb's wool between toes, and properly fitting shoes.

B. The patient should be cautioned about the dangers of excessive hea[t] or cold.

C. Vasodilating drugs are of no proved benefit and need not be prescribed. Consult with physician for patients who are on medicatio[n] previously prescribed by another physician.

D. The patient should avoid cigarette smoking and ingestion of caffein[e].

VII. Complications

A. Gangrene, ulceration.

B. Impaired nail and hair growth.

VIII. Consultation – referral

A. All patients should be discussed with the physician and/or referred within 2 weeks for evaluation regarding further diagnostic studies and consideration for revascularization.

B. Any patient with acute onset of symptoms should be referred that day.

.C. Patients with gangrene or skin ulcers should be referred.

IX. Follow-up

A. All patients should be seen every 3–6 months to follow their circulatory status, and the physician consulted if there is progression of the disease.

B. All patients should be instructed to return if symptoms increase or skin abrasions, lacerations or other breaks in skin surface, inflamma[tion], or infection occurs.

STASIS ULCER OF THE LOWER EXTREMITY (Adult)

I. Definition   A chronic ulcerative lesion of the lower extremity caused [by] poor circulation due to venous stasis.

II. Etiology   Chronic impairment of venous return secondary to varicose veins, a previous episode of thrombophlebitis, or congestive heart failure.

III. Clinical features

A. Symptoms

1. Pain at the site of the ulcer.

2. History of varicose veins or thrombophlebitis.

B. Signs

1. A chronic ulcer of the lower extremity with minimal surrounding inflammation or infection.

2. Associated varicose veins.

3. Usually, pitting edema of the involved leg.

4. Frequently, brawny edema.

5. Negative Homans' sign.

6. Intact peripheral pulses in the involved extremity.

IV. Laboratory studies   None.

V. Differential diagnosis

A. Chronic lymphedema.

B. Arterial occlusive lesion (see Chronic Occlusive Arterial Disease of the Extremities [Adult]).

VI. Treatment

A. Rest and elevation of the involved leg.

B. Muscular activity of elevated leg by such measures as use of a foot board during bed rest.

C. Initial vigorous cleansing of the ulcer by the FNP followed by twice-daily cleansing of the ulcer by the patient at home, using pHisoHex and water, or hydrogen peroxide. Apply dry dressing after cleansing. A pHisoHex soak may be necessary before beginning cleansing.

D. Application of Unna's paste boot if measures **A**–**C** do not result in healing in 3 weeks, particularly if the patient is unable or unwilling to follow the regimen.

VII. Complications

A. Severe extension of ulcer.

B. Cellulitis.

VIII. **Consultation — referral**

A. Surrounding inflammation or infection.

B. Positive Homans' sign.

C. Failure to heal within 1 month.

IX. **Follow-up**   Return visit every 5—7 days until ulcer is healed or consultation is required.

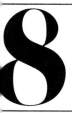

AEROPHAGIA (GASEOUS DISTENTION SYNDROME) (Adult)

 I. **Definition** A syndrome characterized by gaseous distention of the abdomen, which is usually worse after meals and relieved in part by eructation or passage of flatus.

 II. **Etiology** Most of the offending gas is due to air-swallowing. Most of these patients suffer from tension-anxiety states.

III. **Clinical features**

   A. **Symptoms**

     1. Abdominal distention.

     2. Mild, nonlocalized abdominal discomfort.

     3. Eructation and passage of flatus, often with partial relief.

     4. Often, worsening of symptoms just after meals.

     5. No nausea or vomiting.

     6. No change in bowel habits.

   B. **Signs**

     1. No weight loss.

     2. No fever.

     3. Minimal, nonlocalized abdominal tenderness.

     4. Slight to moderate abdominal distention with hyperresonance to percussion.

     5. No fluid wave or shifting dullness.

     6. No masses or visceromegaly.

     7. Normal to slightly hyperactive bowel sounds.

     8. Negative rectal examination.

IV. **Laboratory studies**

    A. Negative stool benzidine test.

    B. Normal hematocrit.

V. **Differential diagnosis**

    A. Intestinal obstruction.

    B. Ascites.

    C. Mesenteric vascular insufficiency.

VI. **Treatment**

    A. Reassurance and explanation of the nature of the problem.

    B. Simethicone (Mylicon), 1 or 2 tablets chewed with each meal.

VII. **Complications**   None.

VIII. **Consultation – referral**   Symptoms persisting more than 4–6 weeks.

IX. **Follow-up**   Return visit if there is no improvement.

CONSTIPATION (Pediatric)

I. **Definition**   Difficulty in passing stools, commonly associated with excessive firmness of stools and a decrease in frequency of defecation.

II. **Etiology**

    A. **Acute constipation** (a change of a few days' to several months' duration from a pattern that was within normal limits)

      1. **Pain on defecation** with secondary retention of stools

        a. Anal fissure.

        b. Anal irritation from diaper dermatitis.

        c. Rarely, perianal abscess.

      2. **Functional causes**

        a. Acute illnesses, especially if associated with decreased appetit and activity, e.g., upper respiratory tract infection in an infan

        b. Uncomfortable circumstances for defecation, e.g., outdoor toilet in cold weather, unfamiliar location of toilet facilities, school where permission is required.

    c. Emotional upset.

    d. Disruption of usual daily routine.

3. **Hard stools**

    a. Drying of stools retained because of the conditions cited in 1 and 2.

    b. Recent change to a constipating diet, e.g., excessive milk products or chocolate and not enough fruits or vegetables or other foods with significant residue.

B. **Chronic constipation**

  1. Psychogenic stool-holding.

  2. Chronic neuromuscular disease.

  3. Aganglionic megacolon (Hirschsprung's disease).

III. **Clinical features**   Depending on the underlying cause, any of the following features may be present:

A. **Symptoms**

  1. **Acute constipation**

    a. Pain on defecation if stool is hard or anal fissure or irritation is present, or both.

    b. Straining on defecation.

    c. Firm stools.

    d. History of blood-tinged stool if anal fissure is present.

    e. Decrease in frequency of defecation from usual pattern.

    f. No vomiting.

    g. Mild abdominal pain, if any.

  2. **Chronic constipation**

    a. **Psychogenic stool-holding**

      (1)   Onset in infancy or early childhood.

      (2)   Huge bowel movements at long intervals.

      (3)   Encopresis.

      (4)   Evidence of behavior problems.

    b. **Aganglionic megacolon**

       (1) Occasionally onset is in newborn period.

       (2) Rare spontaneous passage of formed stool.

       (3) No encopresis. However, "overflow" diarrhea may occu

       (4) Anorexia and vomiting in early infancy.

B. Signs

1. Acute constipation

    a. Physical examination is usually normal.

    b. Anal fissure, marked diaper dermatitis, or perianal abscess ma
be present.

    c. Mild abdominal distention with palpable firm stool is apparen
on abdominal and rectal examination.

2. Chronic constipation

    a. Psychogenic stool-holding

       (1) Rectum is large and filled with soft stool.

       (2) Mild abdominal distention may be present.

       (3) Remainder of physical examination usually renders norr
results.

    b. Aganglionic megacolon

       (1) Rectum usually is empty.

       (2) Abdominal distention with palpable stool masses may
be present.

       (3) Growth may be poor.

IV. Laboratory studies   None.

V. Differential diagnosis

A. Normal patient   Parents may not appreciate or accept the wide
variation of patterns of defecation that are within normal limits.

B. Intestinal obstruction   Abdominal pain and vomiting usually are
present.

VI. Treatment

A. Acute constipation

1. **Treat underlying cause:**

   a. Diaper dermatitis.(see Chapter 3, Diaper Dermatitis).

   b. Anal fissure

      (1) Warm sitz baths.

      (2) Gentle cleansing with soap and water.

      (3) Petrolatum to anus.

      (4) Nonconstipating diet in older children (see 2).

   c. Reassurance if constipation is associated with an acute self-limited illness.

   d. Encouragement of parents to help child avoid or cope with environmental or emotional circumstances that promoted constipation.

2. **Prescribe a nonconstipating diet:**

   a. Add 2 tablespoons of dark corn syrup to 1 quart of infant's milk formula.

   b. Decrease milk intake of older child to less than 1 pint a day.

   c. Increase intake of fresh vegetables, fruit juices, and fruits, especially prunes, raisins, figs, and dates (apples and bananas are least helpful).

3. **Remove fecal impaction,** if present:

   a. Manual removal.

   b. Pediatric Fleet enema.

B. **Chronic constipation**   Consult with physician.

VII. **Complications**

A. **Acute constipation**

   1. Fecal impaction.

   2. Overresponse of parents, with excessive, abnormal concern with and manipulation of child's bowel function, leading to behavior problems, encopresis, stool-holding, and parent-child interaction problems.

B. **Chronic constipation**

   1. Fecal impaction.

     2. Secondary behavior and psychosocial problems.

     3. Failure to thrive and colitis (due to aganglionic megacolon).

VIII. Consultation — referral

    A. Chronic constipation.

    B. Recurrent fecal impaction.

    C. Failure to respond to treatment.

 IX. Follow-up   Return visit if there is no improvement within 1 week.

CONSTIPATION (Adult)

 I. Definition   Properly defined as excessive *hardness* of stool without regard to frequency of bowel movements. Normal frequency of bowel movements can vary greatly, from two or three movements daily to one every 3–5 days; however, a decrease in frequency from the patient usual norm may be significant.

 II. Etiology

    A. Neurotic preoccupation with bowel function rather than true constipation.

    B. Opiates.

    C. Barium following x-ray contrast studies.

    D. Dehydration.

    E. Debilitation in chronically ill persons.

    F. Bed rest.

    G. Colonic cancer.

    H. Hypothyroidism.

III. Clinical features

    A. Symptoms

     1. Increased hardness of stool or difficulty in moving bowels.

     2. Frequency of bowel movement; this is not important if stools are soft and not difficult to pass, unless there has been a recent change in frequency.

     3. Sometimes, abdominal distention.

4. *No abdominal pain* in simple constipation.

5. No nausea or vomiting.

6. No history of blood in stools.

B. **Signs**

1. *No abdominal tenderness* on palpation.

2. Normal bowel sounds. (Absence of bowel sounds does *not* occur in simple constipation.)

3. No hyperactive rushes or tinkles.

4. Sometimes, fecal impaction, particularly in bedridden, debilitated, or elderly patients.

5. Sometimes, palpable fecal material. Feces feel firm, but may be indented. No other intra-abdominal mass may be molded.

IV. **Laboratory and other studies**

A. Stool specimen, if obtained, is negative for occult blood.

B. X-ray or other studies are not indicated for simple constipation.

V. **Differential diagnosis**

A. Failure of bowels to move because of intestinal obstruction or ileus.

B. Hypothyroidism.

VI. **Treatment**

A. Check for the presence of fecal impaction in elderly or debilitated persons. (Remember that fecal impaction often presents as diarrhea.)

B. Increase water intake.

C. Drink warm water or coffee early in the morning to initiate bowel movement.

D. Increase intake of fruits, bulky vegetables, or cereals.

E. If measures **A–D** do not work, try the following medications (start with the milder agents, listed first):

1. Metamucil, 1–2 teaspoons in glass of water 2 or 3 times a day.

2. Milk of magnesia, 15–30 ml before bed (contraindicated in patients with chronic renal disease).

3. Colace, 100 mg twice a day.

F. Use an enema if necessary in preparing constipated patients for sigmoidoscopy or abdominal radiographic studies. Rarely, an enem is necessary for relief of severe constipation in chronically ill person

1. Saline solution, 1–2 liters rectally.

2. Soapsuds, 1–2 liters rectally.

3. Adult Fleet enema.

VII. Complications

A. Hemorrhoids.

B. Rectal fissures.

C. Fecal impaction.

VIII. Consultation – referral

A. Any suspicion of an acute abdominal condition.

B. Abdominal pain or tenderness.

C. Nausea or vomiting associated with failure to move bowels.

D. Hyperactive bowel sounds, or rushes or tinkles.

E. Absence of bowel sounds.

F. Occult blood in stool.

G. Failure to respond to conservative treatment (as outlined in VI).

IX. Follow-up
Patients should be followed until "normal" bowel function resumes, i.e., passage of soft stool without difficulty, since failure to improve may indicate the presence of more serious underlying illness.

SIMPLE DIARRHEA (Adult)

I. Definition
Frequent loose or watery stools that are not bloody, purulent, or fatty in character.

II. Etiology

A. Infections (usually, acute viral infections; less frequently, bacterial and parasitic infections).

B. Psychophysiologic disturbances (often related to stress).

C. Dietary indiscretion.

D. Laxatives.

III. Clinical features

A. Symptoms

1. Frequent loose or watery stools.

2. Sometimes, mild crampy abdominal pain just prior to bowel movement.

3. Absence of gross blood.

4. Epidemiology of current gastrointestinal problems are helpful clue as to etiology.

B. Signs

1. Low-grade or no fever.

2. Slight generalized or no abdominal tenderness. No localized tenderness. No rebound or referred rebound tenderness.

3. Hyperactive bowel sounds.

4. No high-pitched rushes or tinkles.

IV. Laboratory and other studies

A. Stool benzidine test is negative.

B. Studies such as barium enema should be done only after consultation.

C. Stool culture or testing of stool for ova and parasites initially is not necessary.

V. Differential diagnosis

A. Bloody diarrhea

1. Certain infections.

2. Regional enteritis.

3. Ulcerative colitis.

4. Diverticulitis.

5. Certain bowel cancers.

B. **Steatorrhea** Malabsorption syndrome.

VI. Treatment

A. Symptomatic management

1. Kaopectate (kaolin and pectin), 60–90 ml 4 times a day

or

    2. Paregoric, 1 teaspoon orally after each loose stool, not to exceed 6 teaspoons in 24 hours

or

    3. Lomotil (diphenoxylate HCl and atropine sulfate), 1 tablet orally after each loose stool not to exceed 6 tablets in 24 hours (restricted drug).

B. Clear liquid diet of tea, carbonated beverages, or soups until improvement.

VII. Complications

    A. With simple diarrhea, generally none.

    B. With severe diarrhea, dehydration, vascular collapse, or shock.

VIII. Consultation — referral

    A. Bloody stools.

    B. Abdominal tenderness or rebound tenderness.

    C. High fever or toxicity.

    D. Dehydration.

    E. Weight loss greater than 5% of body weight.

    F. Recurrent or chronic diarrhea (diarrhea persisting 5–7 days).

IX. Follow-up   Return visit if no improvement within 48 hours.

FUNCTIONAL BOWEL DISEASE (IRRITABLE COLON SYNDROME) (Adult)

    I. Definition   A syndrome characterized by frequent passage (up to 4–6 movements per day) of small amounts of loose, watery stool associated with mild lower abdominal discomfort and a frequent sensation of a need for further defecation recurring in tense, anxious patients, particularly at times of stress.

    II. Etiology   In some manner, tension and anxiety in susceptible patients produce increased intestinal motility and decreased transit time, leading to frequent loose, watery stool. The bowel itself is not inflamed and appears normal on examination. The disturbance is in bowel function.

III. Clinical features

A. Symptoms

1. Frequent passage (up to 4–6 movements per day) of loose, watery stool.

2. Mild lower abdominal discomfort often preceding and relieved by defecation.

3. No nausea or vomiting.

4. No history of blood in stools. Stools often contain mucus.

B. Signs

1. No weight loss.

2. No fever.

3. Minimal lower abdominal tenderness.

4. No rebound or referred rebound tenderness.

5. Normal to slightly hyperactive bowel sounds.

6. No masses or visceromegaly.

IV. Laboratory studies

A. Stool benzidine test is negative.

B. Hematocrit reading is normal.

C. Stool examination for ova and parasites is negative.

V. Differential diagnosis

A. Inflammatory bowel diseases, e.g., ulcerative colitis and regional enteritis.

B. Infectious causes of diarrhea.

C. Parasitic infestations.

D. Tumors of the large bowel.

VI. Treatment

A. Reassurance as to the nature of the problem.

B. Reduction of stress in life situation.

C. Mild tranquilizer, with physician consultation

    1. Chlordiazepoxide, 10 mg orally 4 times a day.

    2. Diazepam, 5 mg orally 4 times a day.

   D. Antidiarrheal agents: Agents such as paregoric or Lomotil are not indicated.

 VII. **Complications**   None.

VIII. **Consultation – referral**   Failure to improve in 4–6 weeks.

  IX. **Follow-up**   Return visit if no improvement in 3 or 4 days.

ACUTE GASTROENTERITIS (Pediatric)

  I. **Definition**   An acute inflammation of the gastrointestinal tract characterized by passage of stools that are more liquid than normal, usually with an increase from the patient's normal frequency. The disorder is often preceded by or associated with vomiting.

 II. **Etiology**

   A. Usually of **unknown cause** (referred to as *nonspecific gastroenteritis* **or simple diarrhea)**. These may be due to viruses or toxin-producing coliform bacteria.

   B. Occasionally due to the following:

    1. Specific **bacterial infection**

     a. *Shigella* (relatively common in some areas).

     b. *Salmonella.*

    2. Side-effect of **oral antibiotics**, e.g., ampicillin.

    3. **Food poisoning**

     a. *Salmonella.*

     b. Staphylococcal enterotoxin (not an actual infection).

III. **Clinical features**

  A. **Symptoms**

    1. Increased liquid content of stools with no specific color change.

    2. Increased frequency of stools.

    3. Vomiting.

    4. Abdominal pain.

5. Sometimes, coexisting respiratory tract infection or otitis media.

6. Sometimes, flecks of blood in stool as diarrhea continues.

7. With dehydration, listlessness and lethargy.

8. Sometimes, family history of similar illness.

B. **Signs**

1. Sometimes, low-grade fever.

2. Abdominal distention (usually mild).

3. Abdominal tenderness (usually generalized, but may be more prominent in any area).

4. Increased bowel sounds.

5. With dehydration, sunken eyes, dry mucous membranes, decreased skin turgor, and weight loss.

IV. **Laboratory studies**

A. Usually none are necessary.

B. Stool culture for *Shigella* and *Salmonella* should be done if any of the following apply:

1. Blood-tinged mucus in stool.

2. Fever over $102°$ F rectally or $101°$ F orally.

3. Family or closed population outbreak.

4. Diarrhea persisting over several days.

V. **Differential diagnosis**

A. **Normal patient**   Parents may not appreciate or accept the wide variation of patterns of defecation that are within normal limits.

B. **Intussusception**   This usually occurs in a patient aged 3—24 months who has a sudden onset of severe, paroxysmal abdominal pain and vomiting. It may be followed within 8—12 hours by loose stools containing blood and mucus.

C. **Appendicitis**   Rarely, a pelvic appendix can cause diarrhea if appendicitis develops.

VI. **Treatment**

A. **Nonspecific gastroenteritis**

1. Explain to parents that there is no specific therapy to stop symptoms immediately but attention to diet and fluid management (see **3**) is needed. Discourage use of antidiarrheal and antiemetic medications.

2. Search for early signs of dehydration:

   a. Instruct parents to record nature and amount of fluid intake, occurrence of vomiting, the number and character of stools, and frequency of urination.

   b. Weigh the patient carefully at the initial visit and each follow-visit to determine the state of fluid balance. Infants should be weighed naked, and older children, with the same, minimal clothing at each visit.

   c. Examine for sunken eyes, dry mucous membranes, and decreased skin turgor.

3. **Dietary management** of mild diarrhea and vomiting may be varied depending on age (older children are less likely to progress to dehydration and rapidity of improvement:

   a. **First 12 hours**

      (1) Discontinue present diet, including milk.

      (2) Drink small amounts of clear liquids, e.g., cola, ginger ale (at room temperature without carbonation, it may decrease the tendency to vomit), every 2–4 hours.

   b. **Next 12 hours** Increase amounts of clear liquids.

   c. **Next 24 hours**

      (1) If diarrhea has *not* definitely improved, continue with clear liquids. In children under 3 years of age, change to an electrolyte solution (Pedialyte or Lytren). If improvement then results, proceed to step **(2).**

      (2) If diarrhea has definitely improved, add easily absorbed solids to the clear liquid diet, e.g., Jello, salt crackers, or bananas.

   d. If diarrhea continues to improve after 48–72 hours of clear liquids and the simple solid foods listed in **(2)**, the following foods may be gradually added: dry toast, baked potato (without butter), infant cereal mixed with water instead of milk, and more Jell-o.

     e. Milk, cheese, eggs, and fried foods should be withheld until it is certain the foods in **d** are tolerated well.

     f. If milk exacerbates the diarrhea, discontinue it and consult the physician if the patient is a young infant (for whom milk is the major food in the diet).

B. *Shigella* **or** *Salmonella* **gastroenteritis**

    1. Proceed with treatment outlined in **A.**

    2. Consult the physician about the need for specific management, e.g., antibiotic therapy for *Shigella.*

C. Side-effects of oral ampicillin

    1. Diarrhea is usually mild, and ampicillin may be continued unless diarrhea increases.

    2. If diarrhea increases:

      a. Discontinue ampicillin, substituting an alternative antibiotic (consult physician).

      b. Proceed with treatment outlined in **A.**

D. Food poisoning

    1. Proceed with treatment outlined in **A.**

    2. Consult physician about the need for further management, including epidemiologic investigation.

VII. Complications Complications are more likely to occur in infants than in older children:

A. Dehydration.

B. Hypovolemic shock.

C. Inability to tolerate milk during recovery period (probably due to secondary lactase deficiency).

VIII. Consultation – referral

A. Vomiting and diarrhea in children under 3 years of age.

B. Dehydration.

C. Severe abdominal pain.

D. Moderate amount of blood in stools (more than just flecks).

E. Failure to improve with treatment within 48 hours.

F. Inability of a young infant to tolerate return of milk formula to die

G. *Salmonella* or *Shigella* infections or food poisoning.

H. Chronic diarrhea.

IX. **Follow-up**

A. **Under 3 years of age**   Return visit or telephone call daily until improvement occurs.

B. **Over 3 years of age**   Return visit in 48 hours or sooner if there is no improvement.

HIATAL HERNIA WITH ESOPHAGITIS (Adult)

I. **Definition**   Herniation of the stomach through the diaphragm. Hiatal hernia is generally asymptomatic unless associated with esophagitis due to reflux of acid into the esophagus.

II. **Etiology**   Unknown.

III. **Clinical features**

A. **Symptoms**

1. Substernal pain that is worse after meals, after bending over, and at night when lying down.

2. Nausea and vomiting.

3. Benzidine-positive stool. (Hiatal hernia rarely may bleed.)

B. **Signs**   Physical examination is usually normal, but patient may have minimal tenderness on palpation of the epigastrium.

IV. **Laboratory and other studies**

A. Hematocrit determination.

B. Stool benzidine test.

C. Electrocardiogram (if heart disease is suspected).

D. Barium swallow (after consultation with physician).

E. Upper gastrointestinal and gallbladder x-ray series (after consultation with physician).

V. **Differential diagnosis**

A. Strictures (secondary to lye ingestion, carcinoma, stomach tubes).

B. Pains simulating myocardial infarction or other gastrointestinal problems.

C. Peptic ulcer.

D. Esophagitis of other causes.

VI. **Treatment**

A. Frequent feedings.

B. Avoidance of food 2 hours before bedtime.

C. Antacids, 30 cc (1 ounce; 2 tablespoons) 1 hour after meals and just before bedtime.

D. Elevation of head of bed on 6-to-8-inch blocks.

E. Weight reduction.

F. Avoidance of tight clothing around the abdomen and chest.

G. Antispasmodics: These are generally not used.

VII. **Complications**

A. Gastrointestinal bleeding.

B. Anemia.

C. Aspiration.

VIII. **Consultation – referral**

A. Gastrointestinal bleeding.

B. Persistent symptoms.

C. Severe anemia.

D. Weight loss.

E. Difficulty swallowing.

F. Vomiting.

IX. **Follow-up**

A. Monthly clinic check for anemia, gastrointestinal bleeding, and weight loss.

B. Barium swallow and upper gastrointestinal x-ray series, if symptoms change.

UNCOMPLICATED DUODENAL PEPTIC ULCER DISEASE (Adult)

I. **Definition**   Ulceration of duodenal mucosa producing pain. Uncompli
cated peptic ulcer does *not* produce bleeding or obstruction.

II. **Etiology**   The etiology is unknown, but peptic ulceration is related to
some of the following factors:

A. **Neuropsychiatric disorders**

1. Stress.

2. Personality trait.

B. **Endocrine disorders**   (The following conditions are related to increa
hydrochloric acid production.)

1. Hyperparathyroidism.

2. Zollinger-Ellison syndrome.

C. **Drugs**

1. Aspirin.

2. Indomethacin.

3. Reserpine.

4. Phenylbutazone.

5. Steroids.

D. **Other diseases**

1. Cirrhosis.

2. Pancreatitis.

3. Pulmonary disease.

4. Arthritis.

III. **Clinical features**

A. **Symptoms**

1. Abdominal pain (in epigastrium or right upper quadrant) usually
1–2 hours after meals (sooner if gastric ulcer is present).

2. Pain relief with food and antacids.

3. Occurrence of pain at night but not just before breakfast.

      4. Intermittent nausea, vomiting, and belching.

      5. No history of hematemesis or melena.

B. Signs

      1. Direct epigastric tenderness without rebound or referred rebound tenderness.

      2. Normal stool with *no* melena on rectal examination.

IV. Laboratory and other studies

  A. Hematocrit.

  B. Testing of stool for occult blood.

  C. Upper gastrointestinal x-ray series for atypical pain patterns and in males over 45 years with onset of new symptoms.

V. Differential diagnosis

  A. Functional disease.

  B. Hiatal hernia.

  C. Coronary insufficiency.

  D. Gastric ulcer.

  E. Less frequently, mild pancreatitis and biliary colic.

VI. Treatment

  A. Diet: Small frequent feedings. Fats, milk, cream, etc., are not necessary and only increase the risk of atherosclerosis. Avoid caffeine, strong spices, and alcohol.

  B. Antacids, 2 tablespoons (30 cc; 1 ounce) every 2–3 hours while awake.

  C. Anticholinergics: Use only on advice of physician. They are contra-indicated in gastric ulcers, bladder neck obstruction, hiatal hernia, and glaucoma.

  Note Gastric ulcers must be managed differently.

VII. Complications

  A. Gastrointestinal bleeding.

  B. Perforation of the stomach or duodenum and development of peritonitis.

C. Intractable pain.

D. Obstruction.

VIII. Consultation — referral

A. Failure of antacids to relieve symptoms in 2—4 weeks.

B. Gastrointestinal bleeding manifested by melena, occult blood in sto
or a drop in the hematocrit reading of more than 4% even in the
absence of recognized bleeding.

C. Progressive weight loss.

D. Signs and symptoms of an acute abdominal condition, including
rigidity and rebound or referred rebound tenderness.

E. All gastric ulcers.

IX. Follow-up

A. Every 2 weeks for 4 weeks after acute onset of symptoms of pain
(without gastrointestinal bleeding) to check for:

1. Response of pain to antacids.

2. Evidence of gastrointestinal bleeding (history of hematemesis or
melena or benzidine-positive stool).

B. Check for side-effects of antacids, e.g., diarrhea and constipation.
Watch for development of congestive heart failure in elderly patient
if Maalox, Gelusil, or other antacids with high sodium content are
used. (Riopan has a low sodium content.)

C. Watch for side-effects of anticholinergics, e.g., constipation, difficu
in urinating, dry mouth and difficulty in clearing bronchial secretio
and blurred vision.

D. A follow-up upper gastrointestinal series generally is not necessary
for duodenal ulcer that is clinically improved.

E. After 6—8 weeks of effective antacid therapy (relief of symptoms)
antacids may be stopped and regular usage resumed only if symptoms recur.

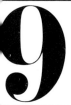

Disorders of the Genitourinary System

CYSTITIS (Adult)

I. **Definition** A condition characterized by inflammation of the bladder, marked by dysuria and frequency, and not usually accompanied by systemic complaints. It is frequently seen in females at the onset of sexual activity.

II. **Etiology**

    A. Bacteria are the most common etiologic agent, and of these, *Escherichia coli* is the most frequently encountered in the ambulatory population. The origin of the bacteria is probably the gastrointestinal tract, and entrance into the urethra is facilitated by sexual activity. Because of the short female urethra, the condition has a predilection for sexually active females.

    B. Occasionally, bacterial pathogens cannot be identified.

III. **Clinical features**

    A. Symptoms

        1. Dysuria, frequency, urgency.

        2. Occasionally, gross hematuria.

        3. Occasionally, low back or lower abdominal pain. No flank or costovertebral pain.

        4. No frank, shaking chills.

        5. Usually, no gastrointestinal complaints.

        6. No vaginal or urethral discharge.

    B. Signs

        1. No fever or temperature less than 101° F.

        2. Only slight lower abdominal tenderness.

        3. No peritoneal signs.

        4. Normal bowel sounds.

        5. No costovertebral angle tenderness.

IV. **Laboratory studies**   Collection of urine for examination is not a casual operation. A clean-catch urine specimen is particularly important for females because of the possibility of vaginal contamination. If epithelial cells appear in a clean-catch urine specimen, the specimen has been contaminated. (See Urinary Tract Infection [Pediatric], **IV.A.1.**)

   A. **Urinalysis**   White and red blood cells and bacteria may be present.

   B. **Urine culture**   A colony count greater than 100,000 of a single urinary tract pathogen generally indicates an infection. (If Gram's stain of unspun sediment is done, the presence of bacteria usually indicates a colony count of greater than 100,000 organisms.)

V. **Differential diagnosis**

   A. **Pyelonephritis**   Patient is usually sick. Although dysuria and frequency are present, these symptoms are overshadowed by systemic complaints of high fever and flank pain; occasional shaking chills occur.

   B. **Vaginitis**   This is associated with vaginal discharge, which may contaminate the urine specimen.

   C. **Urethritis**   Dysuria is usually the chief complaint and generally a discharge, which may be frankly purulent, is present.

   D. **Prostatitis**   Dysuria and frequency may accompany prostatitis, but in acute prostatic infection, systemic symptoms are present and temperature is 100° F. Pain is generally in the lower back and may radiate into the testes.

   E. **Acute abdominal disorder**   Severe abdominal pain and rebound tenderness not found in cystitis are present.

   F. **Cervicitis.**

   G. **Salpingitis.**

VI. **Treatment of initial occurrence**   (Recurrences and reinfection should be referred to a physician.)

   A. **Antibiotics**   Treatment may be instituted with any of the following provided the patient is not allergic to the drug:

   1. **Sulfonamide**   Sulfisoxazole (Gantrisin), 1 gm orally every 6 hours for 10 days after loading dose of 2 gm. In previously untreated cystitis this is the drug of choice. In case of allergy to sulfonamides, use ampicillin (see **2**).

2. **Ampicillin**, 250 mg orally every 6 hours for 10 days.

Note Therapy should be reevaluated when results of culture and sensitivity tests are available, and appropriate changes made if necessary.

B. **Phenazopyridine HCl** (Pyridium), 100 mg orally every 6 hours for 2 or 3 days for bladder analgesic effect, if symptoms warrant. Warn patients that urine will have orange color.

VII. **Complications**

A. Chronic bladder infection.

B. Ascending pyelonephritis.

VIII. **Consultation – referral**

A. Failure to improve in 3 or 4 days.

B. Recurrent cystitis

1. Reinfection within 6 months.

2. More than three episodes over any time span.

C. Growth of original pathogen on follow-up urine culture.

D. All males with cystitis.

IX. **Follow-up** Follow-up urine culture 1 week after treatment course has ended.

ACUTE PYELONEPHRITIS (Adult)

I. **Definition** An infectious disease involving the collecting system and the renal parenchyma of the kidney.

II. **Etiology** Bacterial infection, usually with a gram-negative organism, *Escherichia coli* being the most common.

III. **Clinical features**

A. **Symptoms**

1. Dysuria, frequency, urgency. (These are primarily symptoms of cystitis, but they may be present in pyelonephritis.)

2. Usually, flank pain.

3. Often, frank, shaking chills.

      4. Often, nausea or vomiting, or both.

      5. No vaginal or urethral discharge.

B. Signs

      1. Usually, fever of 101° F or more.

      2. Tenderness on percussion over costovertebral angle.

      3. Negative abdominal examination except for tenderness to deep palpation in the involved flank area.

      4. Patient generally has systemic illness and appears very sick.

IV. Laboratory studies   Use clean-catch urine specimens:

A. Urinalysis shows white blood cells (frequently in clumps), white ce casts, proteinuria, and red blood cells.

B. Urine culture shows a colony count greater than 100,000 of the urinary tract pathogen.

V. Differential diagnosis

A. Cystitis.

B. Prostatitis.

C. Other causes of flank or back pain. (The general public commonly and erroneously considers back pain as tantamount to kidney infection.)

VI. Treatment   The following measures are for an initial occurrence of acute pyelonephritis in an otherwise healthy patient (refer all other patients to a physician):

A. Antibiotics   Ask the patient whether he or she is allergic to the dru

      1. Ampicillin, 500 mg orally every 6 hours for 10 days

        or

      2. Tetracycline, 250 mg orally every 6 hours for 10 days.

B. The patient must be followed closely. If vomiting becomes a comp cation problem, intramuscular medications are necessary.

C. Antibiotics may need to be changed on the basis of clinical response and results of sensitivity testing of the organism.

VII. **Complication**   Chronic pyelonephritis.

VIII. **Consultation — referral**

   A. Severely ill or toxic patient. Patient requiring intramuscular medi--cations.

   B. Diabetics.

   C. Elderly or debilitated patients.

   D. Any recurrence.

   E. Positive culture obtained in follow-up (see **IX.B** and **C**).

IX. **Follow-up**

   A. The patient should be in telephone contact in 24 hours and then every day until asymptomatic.

   B. A repeat urine culture is carried out 1 week after cessation of treatment.

   C. A second repeat culture in about 6 months is desirable.

URINARY TRACT INFECTION (Pediatric)

I. **Definition**   A bacterial infection of the kidneys, collecting system of the kidneys, or bladder, or a combination of these. It includes significant asymptomatic bacteriuria.

II. **Etiology**

   A. Approximately 80% of cases are due to *Escherichia coli.*

   B. The remainder are usually due to *Klebsiella, Proteus mirabilis, Enterobacter, Staphylococcus epidermidis,* enterococci, or *Pseudomonas.*

III. **Clinical features**

   A. **Epidemiology**

      1. **Infants**   Significant bacteriuria is more common in males than females, and has an overall frequency of about 1%.

      2. **Preschool children**   Symptomatic urinary tract infection is relatively common in this age group. Urinary tract infection in general is 10–20 times more common in females than males.

3. **School-age children** Symptomatic urinary tract infection is less frequent than in the preschool period but at least one episode of significant asymptomatic bacteriuria will occur in at least 5–6% of girls between 6 and 17 years of age. The prevalence of asymptomatic bacteriuria is 30 times greater in females. Asymptomatic bacteriuria is associated with increased risk of symptomatic infection in the future.

B. **Symptoms**

1. The infection may be completely asymptomatic and discovered o routine screening for bacteriuria.

2. Urinary tract symptoms may be present:

   a. Urgency, frequency, dysuria.

   b. Enuresis in a child who had achieved control.

   c. Flank pain.

   d. Suprapubic pain.

   e. Foul-smelling or cloudy urine.

   f. Hematuria occasionally in acute cystitis.

3. Various combinations of other symptoms, with or without urinar tract symptoms, may be present:

   a. Gastrointestinal symptoms (i.e., anorexia, nausea, and vomiting).

   b. Abdominal pain.

   c. Lethargy, irritability.

   d. Unexplained fever.

C. **Signs**

1. Sometimes, normal physical examination, and asymptomatic bacteriuria discovered on routine screening.

2. Suprapubic tenderness.

3. Costovertebral angle percussion tenderness.

4. Fever, alone or with other signs and symptoms.

5. Failure to thrive.

IV. Laboratory studies   *The diagnosis of a urinary tract infection is based on the finding of significant growth of bacteria from a urine culture.*

A. Urine culture

1. Collection of specimen[*] (Written instructions[*] should be available for parents, or trained personnel should assist in collecting specimen.)

   a. Urine specimen should be collected in a sterile container after the urethral meatus and surrounding area have been thoroughly sponged with an ordinary liquid soap solution and rinsed with water-soaked sponges. Four soaped sponges followed by four rinse sponges should be used for females. One soaped sponge and one rinse sponge are sufficient for males after the foreskin of uncircumcised males is retracted.

   b. After infancy, a clean-voided *midstream* urine specimen should be collected.

   c. Specimen should be cultured immediately after it is collected. If there is any delay, store specimen in refrigerator.

   d. Drug sensitivity studies for potential urinary pathogens should be requested.

2. Minimal diagnostic criteria

   a. Two consecutive clean-voided specimens revealing 100,000 or more of the same, single urinary pathogen per milliliter of urine are diagnostic.

   b. If only one specimen for culture can be obtained before symptoms require therapy, urinalysis should reveal numerous white blood cells *and* abundant bacteria in order to make a preliminary diagnosis of urinary tract infection.

   c. Lower colony counts (10,000–100,000 organisms per ml) *may* represent infection, especially in patients with recurrent or chronic urinary infections, in patients on suppressive but inadequate antibiotic therapy, and in patients who are emptying their bladders frequently. When the count is between 10,000 and 100,000 organisms per millimeter, culture should be repeated.

[*]For details see Calvin M. Kunin, *Detection, Prevention and Management of Urinary Tract Infections* (2nd ed.). Philadelphia: Lea & Febiger, 1974. Pp. 53–72.

      d. Fewer than 10,000 organisms per milliliter can usually be considered to be contaminants.

      e. Cultures producing colony counts of 100,000 or more per milliliter of mixed organisms should be repeated, as they suggest contamination in a patient who has not had urinary tract instrumentation.

  B. Urinalysis on a clean-voided specimen (examine urine as soon as possible)

    1. Over 20 bacteria per high-power field in the sediment of a centrifuged specimen usually indicate the presence of 100,000 or more organisms per milliliter.

    2. Pyuria *alone* is *not* a reliable guide to the presence of an infection

      a. Pus cells may be contaminants from the vagina and vulva.

      b. Pyuria is absent in up to 50% of patients with significant bacteriuria.

      c. Pyuria may persist for several days after an infection has been successfully treated.

      d. There are other diseases that cause sterile pyuria.

    3. Urine should be examined for other elements — casts, red blood cells, protein, sugar, specific gravity, pH.

V. Differential diagnosis

  A. Vulvovaginitis.

  B. Urethritis.

  C. Prostatitis (in postpuberal male).

  D. Nonbacterial cystitis (e.g., hemorrhage cystitis associated with adeno virus type 11).

VI. Treatment   *Consultation is required before instituting treatment for a urinary tract infection* (see **VIII**). Treatment, after consultation, will usually consist of the following:

  A. Antibiotic   Usually an oral sulfonamide is prescribed for 2 weeks. Be certain the patient is not allergic to the drug. (See Table 5-3 for dosage of sulfisoxazole [Gantrisin] suspension.)

  B. Ample fluid intake and frequent voiding.

VII. Complications

  A. Failure to control infection because organism is resistant to antibiotic prescribed.

  B. Marked systemic toxicity (high fever, vomiting) with possible bacteremia associated with pyelonephritis. Patient may not be able to tolerate oral therapy.

  C. Recurrent infection. In school-age girls, 80% of patients will have at least one recurrence of significant bacteriuria, which may or may not be symptomatic.

  D. Chronic infection, with progressive renal damage. This occurs in very few cases. Patients at risk are usually discovered when radiologic study of the urinary tract is performed.

VIII. Consultation — referral A consultation is required before instituting treatment for a urinary tract infection:

  A. If patient is asymptomatic or only mildly symptomatic, consultation may be requested after the results of the urine cultures are known.

  B. If patient is moderately or markedly symptomatic, consultation should be requested after the results of urinalysis are known.

  C. A consultation is required at the follow-up visit 2 or 3 days after treatment has been started under the following circumstances:

    1. Patient is still symptomatic.

    2. Centrifuged sediment from a clean-voided specimen reveals *bacteria* under high, dry magnification (pyuria may still be present even though infection is being adequately treated).

    3. Urine cultured at follow-up visit is not sterile.

    4. Original urine cultures were not diagnostic of urinary tract infection.

    5. Antibiotic sensitivity studies reveal resistance to prescribed drug.

IX. Follow-up

  A. After 2 or 3 days of therapy

    1. Assessment of clinical status.

    2. Urinalysis on clean-voided specimen.

    3. Urine culture and antibiotic sensitivity testing.

B. If medication is changed at the first follow-up visit, a return visit is again needed in 2 or 3 days for clinical assessment, urinalysis, and urine culture.

C. One week after completing a course of antibiotic therapy

    1. Assessment of clinical status.

    2. Urinalysis on clean-voided specimen.

    3. Urine culture and antibiotic sensitivity testing.

D. *If no further infections occur* the following schedule of visits for clinical assessment, urinalysis, and urine culture are required.

    1. Monthly for 3 consecutive months.

    2. Then every 3 months for the next 9 months.

    3. Then every 6 months for the next year.

    4. Then routine health maintenance visits.

E. Consultation should be requested 6 to 8 weeks after treatment has been completed, concerning the need for an intravenous pyelogram and a voiding cystourethrogram.

GONOCOCCAL URETHRITIS AND VAGINITIS (Adult)

I. Definition   Gonococcal infection of the genitourinary tract.

II. Etiology   *Neisseria gonorrhoeae.*

III. Clinical features

    A. Males   Primary infection may be urethral, pharyngeal, or anorectal.

        1. Occasionally, asymptomatic.

        2. Urethritis (most frequent acute presentation)

            a. Dysuria and frequency.

            b. Purulent discharge.

        3. Pharyngitis from orogenital contact.

        4. Anorectal infection

            a. Anorectal burning.

            b. Mucopurulent discharge.

      c. Painful bowel movements.

  B. Females Primary infection may be urethral, endocervical, pharyngeal, or anorectal.

    1. Occasionally, asymptomatic.

    2. Urethritis: Dysuria, frequency.

    3. Salpingitis

      a. Bilateral lower abdominal pain.

      b. Adnexal tenderness.

      c. Tenderness with manipulation of cervix.

      d. Elevated temperature and chills in some cases.

    4. Pharyngitis from orogenital contact.

    5. Anorectal infection (see **A.4**).

IV. Laboratory studies

  A. Gram's stain of urethral discharge in both male and female.

  B. VDRL test for syphilis.

  C. Culture in cases unproved by Gram's stain. Culture area under suspicion — pharynx, anus, urethra, endocervix. (For urethral culture, insert small swab or wire several centimeters into meatus.) Endocervix is best site for screening in females.

V. Differential diagnosis

  A. Nongonococcal urethritis.

  B. Urinary tract infection.

  C. Acute abdominal disorder (in females), especially those with salpingitis.

  D. Nongonococcal prostatitis.

VI. Prevention

  A. Counsel patients (male and female) concerning use of condoms.

  B. Counsel concerning early treatment of recurrence or reinfection.

  C. Counsel on necessity of contact information in order to prevent further spread of the disease.

VII. Treatment

A. Patients for treatment

1. Patients with urethral discharge showing gram-negative intracell[u] and extracellular diplococci.

2. Patients with known recent exposure to gonorrhea.

3. Patients with positive cultures.

B. Drugs for uncomplicated vaginitis or urethritis[*]

1. Therapy of choice

   a. Probenecid, 1 gm orally followed by b.

   b. Aqueous procaine penicillin, 4.8 million units IM, one-half hour later.

2. Alternative oral therapy (slightly less effective): 3.5 gm ampicil[lin] and 1 gm probenecid at the same time.

3. Therapy in patients allergic to penicillin

   a. Tetracycline HCl, 1.5 gm orally initially, then 0.5 gm orally 4 times a day for 4 days (total, 2.5 gm)

   or

   b. Spectinomycin HCl, 2 gm IM in 1 injection.

C. Instructions to patient

1. Avoid sexual activity for 2 days.

2. Ask sexual contacts to come to clinic for diagnosis and treatme[nt]

VIII. Complications

A. Associated complications

1. Urethral stricture.

2. Rectal stricture.

3. Sterility (infrequent).

B. Infection outside urethra or vagina

1. Salpingitis.

[*]Based on recommendations of the Center for Disease Control, Atlanta, Ga.

2. Pharyngitis (presents as sore throat with exudative pharyngitis).

3. Proctitis.

4. Monoarticular septic arthritis.

5. Disseminated disease.

C. The reappearance of urethral discharge after several days' absence.

IX. Consultation – referral

A. Pharyngitis.

B. Proctitis.

C. Acute abdominal disorder or salpingitis.

D. Tender, swollen adnexa.

E. Fever above 101° F.

F. Arthritis.

G. Rash.

H. Recurrence or positive follow-up culture.

X. Follow-up   Culture in 7–14 days.

A. Males: Urethral culture.

B. Females: Cervical and anal cultures.

XI. Contact and reporting

A. Contact and treat all sexual partners.

B. Report primary case to the health department in the county of residence of the patient.

NONSPECIFIC URETHRITIS (NONGONOCOCCAL URETHRITIS) (Adult)

I. **Definition**   Infection of the urethra not caused by *Neisseria gonorrhoeae.* This syndrome has not been specifically described in females.

II. **Etiology**   *Chlamydia* is felt to be the cause in at least half the cases.[*] In the remainder the cause has not been identified.

---

[*]King K. Holmes. Etiology of nongonococcal urethritis. *N. Engl. J. Med.* 292:1199–1205, 1975.

III. **Clinical features**

    A. **Symptoms**

        1. Dysuria, which is usually not as painful as in gonorrhea.

        2. Increased urinary frequency.

    B. **Signs**   Urethral discharge, which is usually not as copious as in gonorhea and may initially be present only on arising in the morning. The discharge may be milky in appearance and not frankly purulent. This condition may mimic gonorrhea, presenting with extreme dysu and purulent discharge.

IV. **Laboratory studies**

    A. Gram's stain does not reveal gram-negative diplococci.

    B. Gonococcus cannot be cultured.

  V. **Differential diagnosis**   This syndrome must be differentiated from gonococcal urethritis. Although there are some clinical differences, the diagnosis must be established by laboratory findings.

VI. **Treatment**   If Gram's stain does not reveal gram-negative intracellular diplococci, treat with tetracycline, 500 mg every 6 hours for 7 days.

VII. **Complications**

    A. Usually there are no complications.

    B. In a small percentage of patients with a Gram's stain on which no gram-negative intracellular diplococci are found, the culture will be positive.

VIII. **Consultation – referral**   Failure of urethritis to respond to tetracycline

  IX. **Follow-up**

    A. Return visit if symptoms do not improve.

    B. Return visit if culture is positive for *N. gonorrhoeae,* since suggested dose of tetracycline is not sufficient to eradicate gonococcal urethritis.

ACUTE BACTERIAL PROSTATITIS (Adult)

  I. **Definition**   Acute bacterial infection of the prostate gland.

 II. **Etiology**   Usually, *Escherichia coli.* Gonococcus is becoming less common as a cause.

III. **Clinical features**

  A. **Symptoms**

    1. **Local**

      a. Pain in the lower back and perineum, which may be referred into the inguinal area and testes.

      b. Symptoms of urinary obstruction or cystitis, or both.

      c. Tenesmus.

      d. Sometimes, penile discharge that is usually murky white, but may be purulent.

    2. **Systemic**

      a. Fever.

      b. Nausea.

      c. Malaise.

      d. Painful sexual intercourse or frank loss of libido.

  B. **Signs**

    1. Extremely tender, enlarged prostate. Do not massage.

    2. Sometimes, temperature above 101° F.

IV. **Laboratory studies**

  A. Urinalysis usually shows both white and red blood cells.

  B. Urine culture may be positive.

  C. Gram's stain of spun sediment may reveal bacteria.

V. **Differential diagnosis**

  A. Low back pain from muscle strain or chronic prostatitis.

  B. Febrile syndromes (e.g., "flu" syndrome) associated with backache.

VI. **Treatment**

  A. **Antibiotic**   Begin treatment when diagnosis is made – do not wait for results of culture:

    1. Tetracycline, 250–500 mg orally every 6 hours for 10 days

      or

    2. Ampicillin, 500 mg orally every 6 hours for 10 days.

B. **General**

    1. Analgesic for pain.

    2. Sitz bath for 30 minutes 3 times a day.

VII. **Complications**

  A. Chronic bacterial prostatitis.

  B. Urinary retention.

VIII. **Consultation — referral**

  A. No improvement in 3 days.

  B. Recurrence.

  C. Temperature greater than 100° F.

  D. Patient with diabetes mellitus.

  E. Tenderness or swelling of epididymus.

IX. **Follow-up**   Reculture in 3 weeks if initial culture was positive.

PROSTATOSIS (CHRONIC PROSTATITIS)[*] (Adult)

I. **Definition**   A condition of chronic inflammation and congestion of the prostate, not a bacterial infection.

II. **Etiology**

  A. It is not associated with bacteria.

  B. Other infective agents have not been identified.

  C. Perineal trauma may be the initiating event.

III. **Clinical features**

  A. **Symptoms**

    1. Early morning penile discharge.

    2. Vague urinary discomfort, frequently at the termination of micturition.

    3. Dull ache in the perineum, often radiating into the groin or testicles.

[*]Edwin M. Meares. Bacterial prostatitis vs. prostatosis. *J.A.M.A.* 224:1372–1375, 1973.

    4. Diminution of libido.

    5. Low back pain.

  B. Signs The prostate is slightly tender and slightly enlarged; it may be asymmetrical or boggy. Normal landmarks are preserved.

IV. Laboratory studies (Any or all of the following tests may be done and may be helpful in establishing the diagnosis and ruling out infections.)

  A. Urinalysis White blood cells are present in the third glass of a three-glass urine test.

  B. Urine culture is not positive.

  C. Smear of prostatic discharge after massage may contain white cells, but not bacteria.

  D. Culture of prostatic discharge does not produce a pathogenic organism.

V. Differential diagnosis

  A. Acute or chronic bacterial prostatitis.

  B. Other causes of low back pain.

  C. Diseases of the anus, fissure, hemorrhoids.

  D. Cystitis.

VI. Treatment

  A. General

    1. Sitz baths.

    2. Increased sexual activity may help reduce prostatic congestion.

    3. Analgesic for pain.

  B. Local Prostatic massage may decrease congestion.

  C. Antibiotics If culture is positive, treat as bacterial infection (see Acute Bacterial Prostatitis [Adult], **VI.A**).

VII. Complications

  A. Obstruction of urinary outflow.

  B. Chronic pain in the back and groin.

VIII. Consultation – referral

   A. Failure of symptoms to improve after prostatic massage.

   B. Recurrence.

   C. Positive culture.

IX. **Follow-up**   Return visit if symptoms persist.

BENIGN PROSTATIC HYPERTROPHY (Adult)

 I. **Definition**   Hyperplasia of the fibromuscular stroma, with overall enlargement of the gland and compression of the normal prostate tissue.

II. **Etiology**   The cause of benign prostatic hypertrophy is unknown, although the disorder occurs with aging of the male, with symptoms developing in 50% of males over 50 years of age.

III. **Clinical features**

   A. Symptoms

   1. Difficulty in starting micturition.

   2. Difficulty in stopping urine flow.

   3. Small urinary stream.

   4. Small amounts voided each time.

   5. Frequently, nocturia.

   B. Signs

   1. Diffuse enlargement of the prostate gland is present.

   2. No nodules are present. Normal landmarks are preserved.

   3. Bladder may be palpable or percussible above the symphysis pubi because of obstruction.

IV. **Laboratory studies**

   A. Blood urea nitrogen and creatinine levels.

   B. Urinalysis, including microscopic examination.

   C. Urine culture (clean-catch urine specimen).

 V. **Differential diagnosis**

   A. Other causes of obstruction to urinary flow, particularly urethral stricture.

B. Carcinoma of the prostate.

C. Inflammation of the prostate.

D. Other causes of nocturia, e.g., diabetes and congestive heart failure.

> **Note**   In diabetes and congestive heart failure, patients pass large volumes of urine. In benign prostatic hypertrophy, there is frequent, difficult voiding of small amounts of urine.

VI. Treatment   There is no medical treatment for benign prostatic hypertrophy. When symptoms of obstruction occur, the patient must be referred to a urologist for surgical therapy. Because of the prevalence of this disease in elderly males, one must be aware of the potential complications of an enlarged prostate.

VII. Complications

A. Increasing obstruction.

B. Secondary infection.

C. Renal failure.

D. Congestive heart failure. **Note**   In patients with compromised cardiac function, the inability to pass sufficient urine can lead to fluid retention and congestive heart failure.

VIII. Consultation – referral

A. Significant symptoms of obstruction or a palpable or percussible bladder, or both.

B. Acute or symptomatic infection of prostate, or both.

C. Laboratory evidence of decreased renal function.

D. Recurrent urinary tract infection.

IX. Follow-up   Obtain history related to voiding at least once a year, or every visit, if visits occur less frequently than once a year.

VULVOVAGINITIS (Pediatric)

I. Definition   Inflammation of the vulva and vagina, commonly presenting with discharge, pruritus, and erythema.

II. Etiology

A. Nonspecific origin   This type of vulvovaginitis is usually associated with poor hygiene, and no specific microorganism is incriminated.

Culture reveals mixed flora of colonic bacteria (the most common cause in prepuberal females). The inflammation may be aggravated by tight undergarments, especially panty hose or leotards.

B. Irritant

1. Bubble bath (relatively common).

2. Foreign body in vagina (often wads of toilet paper not palpable on rectal examination). Bloody, purulent discharge may ensue.

C. Bacteria

1. Group A beta-hemolytic streptococci (occasionally associated wi scarlet fever).

2. Gonococcus, causing vaginitis in prepuberal females and endo-cervicitis in older females. In infants contamination is from a female caretaker; beyond infancy, suspect sexual contact.

3. Other organisms, including *Staphylococcus aureus* (labial abscess or impetigo causing vulvitis) and *Hemophilus vaginalis* (more common in older females).

D. Parasites

1. Pinworms, which move from the anus into the vagina, where they cause mechanical irritation and scratching.

2. *Trichomonas vaginalis* (common *after* puberty).

E. Fungus   Vulvovaginitis due to *Candida albicans* is common *after* puberty, but occasionally is seen in very young infants, where spread is by hands from vaginitis in an adult.

F. Virus

1. Herpesvirus hominis type 2 usually causes infection in the post-pubertal period (see Chapter 3, Herpes Simplex [Pediatric and Adult]).

2. Vulvovaginitis may be associated with measles or varicella.

III. Clinical features

A. Symptoms

1. Pruritus.

2. Vaginal discharge.

3. Dysuria.

4. Enuresis.

5. Pain with walking or sitting.

6. In a younger child, awkward motions, keeping thighs together while moving, or scratching.

B. Signs

1. Vaginal discharge is usually purulent, and occasionally blood-tinged if a foreign body is present.

2. Excoriations may be present.

3. Erythema of vulva may be present.

4. If poor hygiene is used, one may see bits of stool in the perineal area or pasty, white material between the labial grooves.

5. A foreign body, if hard, may be felt on compression of the vagina during rectal examination.

IV. Laboratory studies

A. Smear of vaginal discharge

1. Obtain a fresh specimen with a cotton swab or dropper after cleansing the vulva.

2. Wet preparation with saline is used to identify *Trichomonas* organisms.

3. Wet preparation with potassium hydroxide is used to detect *Candida* budding yeast with or without hyphae.

4. Gram's stain results are sometimes difficult to interpret because of the large variety of organisms found in the normal prepuberal vagina. Gram's stain is also unreliable for diagnosing gonococcal infection because of the similar appearance of some nonpathogenic organisms.

B. Culture of vulval and vaginal secretions

1. Obtain vaginal specimen by inserting a moist sterile cotton swab after culturing and cleansing the vulva.

2. Order routine bacterial culture.

3. Order gonococcal culture.

Note   The normal prepuberal vagina has a great variety of nonpathoge
bacteria, including *Escherichia coli, Klebsiella,* enterococci, alpha
streptococci, *S. epidermidis, Proteus,* diphtheroids, *Lactobacillus,* and
Pseudomonas.

V. Differential diagnosis

A. Discharge seen normally in first 2 weeks of life (white, nonpurulent
nonodorous, and nonirritating).

B. Discharge seen normally in puberal and immediate prepuberal perio
(asymptomatic and white or mucoid).

VI. Treatment   Treatment is specific, depending on etiology:

A. Discontinue bubble bath.

B. Treat for pinworms if they are seen by a reliable observer (see Chap
ter 15, Pinworms [Pediatric and Adult], **VI**), but **consult also** becau
of the possibility of trapped vaginal pinworms.

C. Treat for specific pathogenic bacteria after review of culture results
and clinical evidence with consultant.

D. See guidelines in Chapter 14 for **candidal vaginitis** and **trichomonal
vaginitis** in postpuberal patients. Since *Trichomonas* may be transmitted venereally, counsel patient appropriately.

E. Use the following measures for **nonspecific vulvovaginitis** and as
general treatment for all patients:

1. Instruct in **perineal hygiene**:

   a. Bathe the perineum gently but carefully with warm water and
   nonperfumed, nonmedicated soap twice a day and after
   defecation.

   b. Remove smegma from between interlabial grooves.

   c. Blot dry — do not rub with a towel.

   d. Then air-dry, with perineum exposed to warm, dry air.

   e. Wear loose, clean, absorbant (cotton) underpants, and
   change them frequently. Do not wear panty hose or leotards.

   f. After defecation, wipe from front to back, with hand coming
   from behind.

   g. Educate child about perineal hygiene if she is old enough.
   Have mother observe child practicing.

2. Take daily **sitz baths** with an acidifying solution (2 tablespoons of vinegar per quart of warm water) to make the vulval and vaginal mucosa less favorable for bacterial growth and provide symptomatic relief.

3. If the vulva is very edematous and tender, apply **cold compresses** of tap water or aluminum acetate (Burow's) solution for 20 minutes 4 times a day.

VII. **Complications** Irritation of the perineum, with development of dermatitis and secondary bacterial skin infection.

VIII. **Consultation – referral**

A. Clinical or laboratory evidence of a bacterial pathogen. Review bacterial culture results with the physician if the organisms are not listed as nonpathogenic in **IV.B. Note.**

B. Pinworm infestation and vulvovaginitis.

C. Suspicion of a foreign body.

D. Failure to respond to treatment within 1 week. These patients will probably need vaginoscopy to rule out a foreign body.

IX. **Follow-up** Return visit in 1 week or sooner if results of culture indicate a need for additional therapy.

ENURESIS (Pediatric)

I. **Definition** Enuresis is an involuntary passage of urine during the day or night. Nocturnal enuresis occurs in about 10–15% of 5-year-olds, 5% of 10-year-olds, and 1% of 15-year-olds.

II. **Etiology**

A. **Unknown cause** This is the most common category. Numerous etiologic theories have been advanced; however, there is no unanimous agreement among authorities. These theories include the following:

1. Psychologic factors.

2. Limited bladder capacity.

3. Delayed neurologic maturation.

4. Profound sleep state.

B. **Variation of normal** Under 5 years of age enuresis can be considered normal unless there are signs and symptoms suggesting a specific cause.

C. Urinary tract infection.

D. Obstructive lesions of the urinary tract.

E. Primary neurologic disorder.

F. Disorders associated with **decreased urine-concentrating ability and increased volume,** causing enuresis.

III. Clinical features

A. Symptoms

1. The passage of urine may occur from rarely to several times daily, day or night. In children, who have achieved good control, there may be periodic lapses at night for several years.

2. Boys are affected somewhat more frequently than girls.

3. There is a familial tendency.

B. Signs   Results of a complete physical examination are usually normal; however, particular attention should be paid to the following:

1. Evidence of psychologic and behavior problems.

2. Lumbosacral skin abnormalities.

3. Abnormalities of the genitalia, including the urethral meatus.

4. Poor rectal sphincter tone.

5. Decreased perineal sensation to pinprick.

IV. Laboratory studies

A. Urinalysis and measurement of specific gravity (ideally on a first morning specimen to assess concentrating ability).

B. Urine culture (see Urinary Tract Infection [Pediatric], **IV.A,** for technique and interpretation).

V. Differential diagnosis   None.

VI. Treatment

A. General counseling

1. Reassurance for children under 5 years of age that enuresis is still

normal at that age unless symptoms or signs suggest a specific cause.

2. Avoidance of punishment or ridicule for enuresis, as it is not voluntary. Secondary psychologic problems can result if enuresis is managed inappropriately by the family.

3. Reassurance that even if nothing is done, enuresis is most often a self-limited condition if there is no specific underlying cause that can be found.

B. **Therapy for children over 5 years of age** (after examination and laboratory studies reveal no specific cause)

1. Have patient keep a diary of wet and dry days and nights for 1 month.

2. If daytime enuresis occurs, consult physician.

3. If only nocturnal enuresis occurs, suggest the following measures. (The efficacy of these suggestions has not been proved, but each has the support of some clinicians.)

   a. Limit fluid intake after evening meal.

   b. Suggest that before the parents go to bed, they awaken the child to urinate.

   c. Encourage the child to become involved in the therapeutic process:

      (1) Have the patient keep a diary of wet and dry nights.

      (2) Have him set an alarm clock to allow urination during the night. Sleep intervals may gradually be lengthened.

      (3) Suggest that the patient retain urine for progressively longer periods during the day.

   d. Schedule return visit in 1 month.

   e. If enuresis has not decreased, consult the physician.

   f. If enuresis has decreased, give praise and continue to see the patient periodically on the basis of degree of improvement and need for counseling.

VII. **Complications**   Secondary psychologic problems because of:

   A. Punitive or ridiculing family attitude.

    B. Inability of child to participate in certain social activities, e.g., camp and overnight visits.

VIII. Consultation — referral

    A. Daytime enuresis.

    B. Evidence suggesting specific organic cause.

    C. Severe psychologic problems.

    D. Failure to improve after treatment.

IX. Follow-up   See **VI.B.3.d–f.**

10 Disorders of the Musculoskeletal System

MINOR ANKLE SPRAIN (Pediatric and Adult)

I. Definition An injury to the ankle resulting in stretching of the ligament. In a mild sprain, there is no tear of the ligament.

II. Etiology Sprain is most often due to inversion-plantar flexion injury ("I rolled my ankle over").

II. Clinical features

A. Symptoms

1. Pain over the lateral aspect of the ankle.

2. Patient did *not* hear or feel a "pop" or "snap" at the time of injury. (A "pop" or "snap" suggests a ligamental tear or fracture.)

B. Signs

1. *No* ecchymoses.

2. Minimal, somewhat diffuse tenderness over the medial or lateral malleolus.

3. *No* focal area of exquisite tenderness.

4. Minimal or *no* swelling.

5. No instability of joint.

V. Diagnostic studies With mild injury, x-ray films are not indicated.

V. Differential diagnosis

A. Ligamental tears.

B. Fractures.

I. Treatment

A. Keep weight off the ankle, with either bed rest or use of crutches.

B. Wrap ankle with Ace bandage.

C. Apply an ice pack to the ankle for the first 24 hours to prevent swelling.

D. Follow with heat to the ankle, if necessary.

VII. **Complications**   None with minor sprain.

VIII. **Consultation – referral**

A. All sprains associated with ecchymoses, focal or moderate to severe tenderness, more than minimal swelling, or instability of a joint.

B. All possible fractures.

IX. **Follow-up**   Return visit in 24 hours; if the sprain is not significantly improved, refer for x-ray study and consultation.

MINOR STRAINS AND SPRAINS* (Pediatric and Adult)

I. **Definition**   Minor injury to a joint where the nature of the trauma was mild, resulting in minimal stretching of the involved ligaments and contusion of the surrounding soft tissues.

II. **Etiology**   Strains and sprains usually result from a fall, a blow from another person, or an automobile accident. In cases to be managed by the FNP, the history of the nature of the injury should suggest only minor trauma, for example, falling on the ground, a child's receiving a blow from another child, or a minor automobile accident. Although minor trauma does not ensure that the injury is not severe, it is an important point to note. All cases involving major trauma, such as severe automobile accidents, should *not* be managed by the FNP.

III. **Clinical features**

A. **Symptoms**

1. Mild pain around the site of injury.

2. Minimal or no loss of function of the involved area.

B. **Signs**

1. *No* ecchymoses.

2. *No* instability.

3. *No* focal tenderness over the involved ligaments or bones.

4. *No* crepitance.

*Excluding ankle sprains. For these, see Minor Ankle Sprain (Pediatric and Adult).

      5. *Minimal* or *no* swelling of the involved area.

IV. **Diagnostic studies** X-ray films are not indicated in minor injuries.

V. **Differential diagnosis**

  A. Severe sprain with or without fracture, suggested by the following symptoms:

    1. Severe pain.

    2. Loss of function.

    3. Ecchymoses.

    4. Point tenderness.

    5. Instability.

    6. Crepitance.

    7. Moderate or severe swelling.

  B. Fractures.

VI. **Treatment**

  A. Immobilization of joint for 24–36 hours.

  B. Ice pack for 24 hours.

  C. Local heat after first 24 hours, if needed.

VII. **Complications** None.

VIII. **Consultation – referral** All injuries associated with:

  A. Ecchymoses.

  B. Focal or moderate to severe tenderness.

  C. More than minimal swelling.

  D. Instability of the joint.

IX. **Follow-up** A return visit is mandatory if there is *no* improvement in 24 hours or incomplete resolution in 1 week.

MUSCULOSKELETAL CHEST PAIN (Adult)

I. **Definition** Pain in the chest arising from (1) the bony structures of the rib cage and associated upper-limb girdle, (2) the skeletal muscle related to the chest and upper limb, or (3) a combination of these.

II. **Etiology**   The pain frequently is related to unusual muscular exertion involving the upper limb or chest, or both. Trauma may be implicated. In many cases, the cause is unknown.

III. **Clinical features**

A. **Symptoms**

1. The pain is usually aggravated by activity producing either movement of the chest cage or upper extremity or pressure on the chest or both, and relieved by rest or release of pressure.

2. The pain is *not produced by general exertion,* such as walking up a flight of stairs, or other exertion not requiring movement of the chest or arm.

3. The pain often occurs late in the day after the patient has indulged in strenuous exertion involving the chest or arm.

4. The pain is frequently described as sharp, momentary, and stable.

B. **Signs**

1. Pain is often reproduced by either movement of the arm or chest or pressure on the chest cage or muscles involved, or both.

2. The chest is clear on auscultation.

3. Cardiac examination is normal.

IV. **Diagnostic studies**

A. Seldom indicated.

B. Electrocardiography may be done in older patients for reassurance. One should not rely on it to make a diagnosis, however.

V. **Differential diagnosis**

A. Angina pectoris.

B. Myocardial infarction.

C. Pleuritic chest pain.

D. Esophagitis and other gastrointestinal causes of chest pain.

E. Cervical spine disease (disk disease and osteophytosis produce nerve root compression).

VI. **Treatment**

A. Reassurance as to the origin of the pain.

B. Heat on the involved area.

C. Rest.

D. Aspirin (325 mg per tablet), 1 or 2 tablets orally every 4–6 hours.

VII. Complications These are primarily psychological, relating to the patient's concern that the pain is cardiac in origin.

III. Consultation – referral

A. Unclear diagnosis.

B. Unusual patient anxiety even if the diagnosis seems readily apparent.

IX. Follow-up As needed for the reassurance of both the patient and the FNP.

LUMBOSACRAL STRAIN (Adult)

I. Definition A painful condition involving the lower back. It is usually chronic, with acute exacerbations often related to physical stress.

II. Etiology Pain arises from strain of the ligaments and musculature of the lumbosacral area, and not from the spine, articular cartilage, or nerve roots.

III. Clinical features

A. Symptoms

1. Usually mild to moderately severe pain located across the lumbosacral area, generally worsened by movement, as getting out of bed, rising from a sitting position, or bending over.

2. No radicular pain.

3. No radiation of pain to legs, groin, or testes.

4. No costovertebral angle pain.

5. No dysuria, frequency, or other genitourinary symptoms.

B. Signs

1. No fever.

2. Pain and muscle spasm on palpation over lumbosacral area.

3. No pain in flanks on percussion.

4. Minimal or no pain on straight leg raising.

    5. Normal neurologic examination of lower extremities, including sensory and motor function and reflexes.

    6. Intact pulses in lower extremities.

IV. **Diagnostic studies**   None.

V. **Differential diagnosis**

    A. Lumbosacral disk disease.

    B. Genitourinary infections, including cystitis, prostatitis, and pyelonephritis.

    C. Vascular occlusion at the level of the aortic bifurcation.

    D. Cancer with bony metastases (cancer of the prostate often presents in this manner).

    E. Gynecologic disorders, e.g., endometriosis and fibromyomas.

VI. **Treatment**

    A. For moderately severe pain, bedrest. For minimal pain, restriction of activity, particularly lifting.

    B. Bed board.

    C. Aspirin, 1 or 2 tablets (325 mg per tablet) orally every 4–6 hours.

    D. Local heat.

VII. **Complications**   Prolonged disability that is probably due to a combination of physical, psychologic, social, and economic factors.

VIII. **Consultation – referral**

    A. Severe, disabling pain.

    B. Prolonged pain (lasting more than 2 weeks).

    C. Recurrent pain (more than three attacks).

IX. **Follow-up**   Return visit if there is no improvement within several days

NONSPECIFIC MUSCULOSKELETAL PAIN (Adult)

I. **Definition**   Vague aching of the muscles, bones, joints, or ligaments (alone or in any combination), usually poorly localized to areas such as the arm and shoulder, the hip and leg, and the anterior chest and arm.

II. Etiology

A. Trauma or straining of the involved area by excessive use is often implicated.

B. Frequently no obvious cause can be ascertained.

C. Nonspecific musculoskeletal pain is often associated with tension-anxiety states.

III. Clinical features

A. Symptoms

1. A vague aching of the muscles, bones, joints, or ligaments, usually poorly localized to areas such as the arm and shoulder, the hip and leg, and the anterior chest and arm.

2. *No* generalized myalgia.

3. *No* localized musculoskeletal pain as in bursitis or arthritis.

4. *No* neurologic symptoms such as sensory loss or localized weakness.

5. Sometimes, history of trauma to or excessive or unusual use of the involved area.

B. Signs

1. No fever.

2. No objective inflammation, i.e., no redness, swelling, heat, or warmth of any part of the painful area.

3. No demonstrable sensory or motor deficit.

4. Sometimes, vague, poorly localized tenderness to palpation of the involved muscles, joints, ligaments, or bones.

IV. Diagnostic studies   None.

V. Differential diagnosis

A. Specific localized inflammatory conditions affecting the musculoskeletal system, e.g., arthritis, bursitis, tendinitis, and gout.

B. Generalized myalgia accompanying systemic illnesses, e.g., influenza, Rocky Mountain spotted fever, and pneumonia.

C. Specific localized symptoms related to known trauma, e.g., sprained ankle.

VI. **Treatment**

    A. Rest of the involved area.

    B. Heat by means of a hot water bottle, heating pad, warm soaks, hot showers, etc.

    C. Aspirin (325 mg per tablet), 2 tablets taken orally every 4–6 hours.

VII. **Complications**   Prolonged disability.

VIII. **Consultation – referral**

    A. Severe pain.

    B. Course prolonged more than 2 weeks.

    C. Recurrent pain (more than three attacks).

IX. **Follow-up**   As needed.

OSTEOARTHRITIS (Adult)

I. **Definition**   A disorder usually restricted to elderly people and characized by degeneration of articular cartilage and hypertrophy of bone, usually in weight-bearing joints and in the distal interphalangeal joints of the fingers.

II. **Etiology**   Osteoarthritis is associated with aging and trauma, but no specific cause has been found.

III. **Clinical features**

    A. **Symptoms**

        1. Joint pain and stiffness are present. The pain characteristically improves with rest and worsens with exercise, while the stiffness improves with exercise.

        2. Pain is usually mild and rarely progresses to the point of invalidi although the affected fingers may become difficult to move easi and with precision.

        3. Cervical lesions may lead to neck pain and may cause radicular neuropathy, with pain and weakness in the arm or the shoulder girdle.

    B. **Signs**

        1. The joints most commonly affected are the knees, hips, lumbar

vertebrae (weight-bearing joints), cervical vertebrae, and distal interphalangeal joints of the fingers.

2. Affected joints are not hot or erythematous, but may be mildly tender.

3. Classically, interphalangeal involvement leads to Heberden's nodes, firm, knotty enlargements of the distal interphalangeal joints, which may be present alone without other joint involvement.

4. Larger joints and vertebrae usually appear grossly normal.

IV. Laboratory and other studies

A. An x-ray film of the involved joint is useful if the diagnosis is in question. (Heberden's nodes do not require x-ray.)

B. Determination of the sedimentation rate also may be helpful to establish the presence or absence of an inflammatory process.

V. Differential diagnosis

A. Polyarthritis

1. Acute rheumatoid arthritis is usually easily differentiated because the affected joints are inflamed, there may be constitutional signs and symptoms, and the sedimentation rate is elevated.

2. Chronic rheumatoid arthritis affects the proximal interphalangeal and the metacarpal phalangeal joints.

3. In addition to bone involvement, there is swelling of synovial tissue and edema around the joints in both acute and chronic rheumatoid arthritis.

B. Monarticular arthritis

1. Gout (see Chapter 12, Gout and Hyperuricemia [Adult]).

2. Traumatic arthritis: Generally the joints are swollen and tender and there is a history of trauma.

3. Infection: Inflammatory arthritis is frequently associated with gonococcal infection occurring in a much younger age group.

Note Osteoarthritis may be present along with an inflammatory arthritis. If the degree of pain and inflammation seems incompatible with osteoarthritis, one should seek another cause.

VI. Treatment

A. Rest of the involved joints.

B. Physical therapy of the joints.

C. Aspirin for pain, 1 or 2 tablets (325 mg) every 4–6 hours.

D. Heat to the involved joints.

E. Weight loss and elimination of trauma.

F. In some cases, a neck or back support.

VII. **Complications**

A. Generally osteoarthritis is not severe or crippling and usually results in no systemic complaints.

B. Cervical vertebral lesions occasionally lead to radicular neurologic problems.

VIII. **Consultation — referral**

A. Inflammatory arthritis.

B. Neurologic involvement.

IX. **Follow-up**

A. These patients may be seen as needed for exacerbation of pain or dysfunction.

B. Special visits generally are not necessary; the osteoarthritis may be evaluated during visits for other problems or for health maintenance.

DIZZINESS IN ADULTS LESS THAN 50 YEARS OLD

I. **Definition** A vague sensation of unsteadiness or lightheadedness, or both, occurring episodically in adults less than 50 years old.

II. **Etiology** Most often seen in association with tension-anxiety states.

II. **Clinical features**

A. **Symptoms**

1. A vague sensation of unsteadiness, as though one might fall in one direction or another.

2. No vertigo.

3. No tendency to fall consistently in one direction.

4. No associated severe headache.

5. No associated neurologic symptoms.

6. No associated nausea or vomiting.

7. Feeling of faintness or a sensation of loss of consciousness, but no actual loss of consciousness.

8. Attacks not precipitated by prior ingestion (1–1½ hours before attack) of heavy carbohydrate meal or relieved by ingestion of food.

B. **Signs**

1. Blood pressure between 100/70 and 150/100 mm Hg, with orthostatic drop of less than 10 mm Hg diastolic.

2. Normal neurologic examination.

3. No murmur of aortic stenosis.

V. **Laboratory studies** Hematocrit reading is normal.

V. **Differential diagnosis**

A. Vasovagal syncope.

B. Vertiginous dizziness, as in labyrinthitis, Meniere's syndrome, and acoustic neuroma.

C. Postural hypotension, especially in patients being treated for hype
tension.

D. Acute blood loss, as in gastrointestinal hemorrhage.

E. Unsteadiness associated with significant anemia (hematocrit readin
less than 35%).

F. Dizziness associated with aortic stenosis.

G. Dizziness associated with other neurologic symptoms or signs, as i
stroke syndrome.

H. Hypoglycemic episodes.

VI. **Treatment**

A. Reassurance as to the absence of serious disease.

B. Attempts to discover and alter psychosocial factors that often are
associated.

VII. **Complications**   Prolonged disability.

VIII. **Consultation – referral**   Severe, persistent (single attack lasting more
24 hours), or recurring (more than six per week) attacks.

IX. **Follow-up**   As needed.

MIGRAINE HEADACHE (Adult)

I. **Definition**   A throbbing unilateral headache with familial tendency t
is preceded by an aura and by other neurologic manifestations in mar
cases.

II. **Etiology**   Unknown. Pain is related to cerebral arterial spasm follow
by dilation. It is during the dilation phase that pain occurs.

III. **Clinical features**

A. Headache is usually unilateral, but not always on the same side.

B. Headaches are generally preceded by a visual aura, which may be
followed by neurologic signs, such as tingling and weakness in an
extremity. There may actually be temporary paralysis.

C. Throbbing gradually increases in intensity to a peak in 1 hour and
then may last for a few hours to several days. It may be associated
with nausea and vomiting.

D. Photophobia may be present.

    E. Eighty percent of patients have a family history of migraine.

    F. Onset is generally in adolescence and attacks tend to decrease in frequency with age. However, migraine may begin at a later age and actually accelerate in frequency in menopause.

IV. Laboratory studies   None.

V. Differential diagnosis   See Tension Headache (Adult), **V.**

VI. Treatment

    A. At the first sign of headache, use either of the following:

        1. Ergotrate (ergonovine) maleate, 3 mg sublingually initially, followed by 2 mg every one-half hour until headache is relieved (to a total of 9 mg).

        2. Cafergot (ergotamine tartrate and caffeine), 2 tablets initially, followed by a third in one-half hour. This may also be taken as a rectal suppository (2 mg ergotamine and 100 mg caffeine) if vomiting precludes oral administration.

    B. In established headache, an ergot preparation may be tried (see **A**), but generally the following measures are required:

        1. Dark room.

        2. Analgesic, such as codeine or meperidine HCl (Demerol). Both are controlled medicines requiring physician's orders.

    C. Preventive treatment with methysergide maleate (Sansert) is carried out under the physician's direction. **Note**   Retroperitoneal fibrosis has been reported in patients on methysergide.

VII. Complications   Generally, there are no complications.

VIII. Consultation – referral

    A. Failure of treatment.

    B. All new cases (first time to clinic or first time with headache).

    C. Persistence of neurologic component.

IX. Follow-up   Return visit if there is no improvement.

TENSION HEADACHE (Adult)

    I. Definition   A headache generally associated with periods of stress that is characterized by a bandlike pressure across the forehead and occiput.

II. Etiology   The headache is generally associated with tension, but the cause is not specifically known. Pain may be associated with muscle spasm.

III. Clinical features

   A. Symptoms

   1. Dull, aching pain occurs bilaterally across the scalp.

   2. Usually middle-aged persons are affected.

   3. Headache is present for long periods of time.

   4. Pain is not throbbing.

   5. Associated nausea and vomiting generally are not present.

   6. Headache may be associated with known periods of tension.

   7. No aura or neurologic deficit is present.

   B. Signs

   1. Generally there are no signs:

      a. Blood pressure is normal.

      b. Results of funduscopic examination are normal; pupils are reactive.

      c. Results of the screening neurologic examination are normal.

      d. No febrile disease is present.

      e. The temporal arteries are nontender.

   2. The scalp may be sore.

   3. The muscles in the posterior neck may be tense and tender.

IV. Laboratory studies   None.

V. Differential diagnosis   Eliminate other major causes of headache.

   A. Sinus headache   Pain is located over antrum, forehead, or around the eyes, most frequently in association with sinus congestion but sometimes in association with bacterial sinusitis. The overlying skin may be sensitive and the sinuses tender. Headache may begin at night and change sides with change in position.

B. Migraine   See Migraine Headache (Adult).

C. Hypertension   Hypertension may cause early morning headaches, but moderate hypertension does not usually cause significantly severe headaches.

D. Systemic febrile disease.

E. Glaucoma   Pain is generally severe and is located around the orbits. It may be associated with nausea and vomiting. Pupils are fixed and semidilated.

F. Brain tumor   Headache associated with brain tumor does not have a specific character but tends to be a more severe, deep-seated pain that may come and go and tends to worsen. It may occur at night and wake the patient; it may also occur in the early morning.

G. Cluster headache (Horton's headache)   Cluster headache occurs generally at night, is generally localized to one orbit, and lasts approximately 1 hour. Intense pain associated with rhinorrhea, lacrimation, and flush is present. The pains tend to occur in clusters over a period of a few nights to weeks and then disappear.

VI. Treatment

A. Reassurance.

B. Analgesic — aspirin, 1 or 2 tablets (325 mg) every 6 hours.

C. If stress is identifiable, a mild tranquilizer may be added on physician's advice.

VII. Complications   Rare.

VIII. Consultation — referral

A. Tension headache that does not improve after initial therapy has begun.

B. All headaches not specifically diagnosed as migraine, sinus, or mild headache associated with hypertension. Failure to resolve after 2 weeks of treatment.

IX. Follow-up

A. Return visit in 2 weeks, or sooner if necessary

or

B. Allow patient to initiate next visit.

VASOVAGAL SYNCOPE (SIMPLE FAINT)
IN ADULTS LESS THAN 60 YEARS OLD

I. **Definition** A transient loss of consciousness and motor function due to a transient, reversible decrease in general cerebral blood flow.

II. **Etiology** Vasovagal syncope is the result of a complex phenomenon involving, in part, vagal nerve stimulation with resultant bradycardia and venous pooling of blood in the extremities and viscera. It is often triggered by emotional factors, such as venipuncture or disturbing news. The cardiovascular phenomena are transient in nature, lasting only a few minutes.

III. **Clinical features**

A. **Symptoms**

1. Loss of consciousness preceded by a *sensation of faintness often associated with slight nausea and mild diaphoresis.*

2. No headache or localizing neurologic symptoms.

3. Prompt return of consciousness, with no postictal state.

4. No history of organic heart disease, such as angina or arrhythmia.

B. **Signs**

1. Weak, thready pulse, often with bradycardia.

2. Blood pressure during actual faint often less than 70 mm Hg systolic.

3. Pallor.

4. Diaphoresis.

5. Sometimes, twitching of extremities, but no definite seizure activity.

6. No bladder or bowel incontinence.

7. No postictal confusion.

8. No demonstrable neurologic deficit in postfaint evaluation.

9. No murmur of aortic stenosis.

IV. **Laboratory studies** None.

V. **Differential diagnosis**

    A. Grand mal or other seizure disorder.

    B. Localized transient cerebral ischemia, as in stroke syndromes.

    C. Syncope occurring with aortic stenosis.

    D. Syncope occurring with tachycardia or bradycardia associated with organic heart disease.

VI. Treatment

    A. Position patient so that his head is lower than his feet, or simply place him supine on the floor or ground.

    B. Record blood pressure and pulse every 5 minutes.

    C. Obtain an electrocardiogram if pulse is irregular.

VII. Complications　None.

VIII. Consultation – referral

    A. Convulsion.

    B. Presence of any abnormal neurologic finding.

    C. Patient over 60 years of age.

    D. Orthostatic fall in blood pressure.

    E. Hematocrit reading below normal.

    F. Melena.

    G. Murmur of aortic stenosis.

    H. Abnormal pulse.

    I. Failure of blood pressure and pulse to return to normal in 15 minutes.

IX. Follow-up　As needed.

ANXIETY (Adult)

I. Definition　State of apprehension, restlessness, nervousness, or fearfulness, which can be longstanding or relatively acute.

II. Etiology

    A. Life situations, usually associated with a family or personal crisis.

    B. Certain physical and mental illnesses.

III. Clinical features

A. Symptoms

1. Anorexia, insomnia, increased sweating, thumping in the heart, irritability, weakness and fatigue, and headaches.

2. Weight loss, nausea and vomiting, diarrhea, numbness and tingling of extremities, shortness of breath, polyuria, and amenorrhea indicate complications other than, or in addition to, simple anxiety.

B. Signs

1. Trembling of fingers, increased sweating, drawn face and tight muscles, and tachycardia.

2. Weight loss, slow speech, and flat affect indicate complications other than, or in addition to, simple anxiety.

IV. Laboratory studies   None.

V. Differential diagnosis

A. Hyperthyroidism.

B. Cancer.

C. Organic brain syndrome.

D. Unexplained weight loss due to other causes.

E. Hypertension.

F. Depression.

G. Alcoholism.

H. Drug abuse.

VI. Treatment

A. Supportive therapy using supportive staff as much as possible and/or frequent *short* visits to health center.

B. Diazepam (Valium), 2–5 mg orally 3 or 4 times a day for a maximum of 2 weeks.

C. If patient is elderly or demonstrates organic brain changes, chlorpromazine (Thorazine) or thioridazine (Mellaril), 10 mg orally up to 4 times a day, should be substituted for Valium for a maximum of 2 weeks (consultation required).

   D. Contraindications to drug therapy include:

   1. First trimester of pregnancy.

   2. Grief reactions: Nighttime sedation is appropriate, but tranquilization is not.

   3. Active liver disease.

   4. History of agranulocytosis (phenothiazines contraindicated).

   5. Suspected drug abuse: If acute withdrawal is suspected, hospitalization is indicated.

   6. Glaucoma.

VII. Complications

   A. Drug abuse.

   B. Psychoactive drugs should be used only after consultation, and in reduced dosage, in patients with impaired renal function.

   C. Valium

   1. **Oversedation**   Patient should be warned that driving may be hazardous and should be urged to start drugs at time when he or she has no responsibility for driving, operating heavy machinery, and so on. If patient appears intoxicated, drug dose should be decreased.

   2. **Potentiating effect**   Valium has a potentiating effect with other depressants, tranquilizers, and narcotics; if patient is undergoing treatment with such drugs, use of depressants should be avoided and consultation sought.

   3. **Confusion and agitation**   These complications may occur in the elderly with depressant drug treatment. Discontinue Valium immediately if confusion or agitation occurs.

   D. Mellaril/Thorazine

   1. **Oversedation**   See C.1.

   2. **Orthostatic hypotension**   Obtain consultation before instituting phenothiazine treatment in a patient with unstable cardiovascular status (e.g., recent myocardial infarction or cerebrovascular accident).

VIII. Consultation – referral

A. Evidence of underlying organic or other disease state, including manifestation of any of the symptoms or signs indicated as *not* consistent with simple anxiety (see **III.A** and **B**).

B. All elderly patients before prescribing Thorazine or Mellaril.

C. Mental health referral is indicated if:

1. There is evidence of depressant drug abuse, e.g., concurrent use of other depressants, such as Librium, barbiturates, or alcohol. Often such a patient demands drugs but gives an unclear or vague history, which is judged to be unreliable.

2. There is evidence by history that the presenting symptoms are of a longstanding nature and have not been precipitated by a real life crisis.

3. At the end of 2 weeks of treatment symptoms persist and the patient requires continued treatment with tranquilizers.

IX. Follow-up

A. Return visit in 2 weeks if medication is prescribed.

B. Return visits as often as necessary, depending on severity of problem and need for ongoing supportive therapy.

Disorders of the Endocrine System

DIABETES MELLITUS (Adult)

I. **Definition** Diabetes mellitus is probably an inherited disease, and it is characterized by two components:

   A. A metabolic component whose major manifestation is elevation of the blood glucose level.

   B. A vascular component, leading in some patients to accelerated athero-sclerosis that affects the small blood vessels, particularly the eyes, kidneys, and nerves.

II. **Etiology** See I.

III. **Clinical features**

   A. **Symptoms**

   1. Symptoms related to high blood glucose levels

      a. Polyuria.

      b. Polydipsia.

      c. Polyphagia.

      d. Weight loss.

      e. Blurred vision secondary to elevated glucose level in the aqueous humor of the eye.

   2. Symptoms related to vascular complications

      a. Eyes: Gradual diminution of vision.

      b. Kidneys

         (1) Edema.

         (2) Eventually symptoms of uremia.

      c. Nervous system

         (1) Paresthesia.

         (2) Numbness.

   (3) Weakness.

   (4) Symptoms of disturbed autonomic function (orthostat hypotension, diarrhea, bladder difficulty, impotence).

  d. Heart: Symptoms of arteriosclerotic heart disease.

  e. Peripheral vascular disease

   (1) Cool extremities.

   (2) Claudication.

 3. Other common symptoms

  a. Vaginal itching, usually secondary to candidal infection.

  b. Skin infections.

B. Signs

 1. Microaneurysms, hemorrhages, and exudates in ocular fundus.

 2. Evidence of advanced atherosclerosis

  a. Coronary heart disease.

  b. Vascular insufficiency in the feet

   (1) Poor pulses.

   (2) Bruits.

   (3) Ulcers.

   (4) Gangrene.

  c. Lowered capillary filling.

 3. Evidence of nervous system dysfunction

  a. Absent knee-ankle jerks.

  b. Areas of sensory loss, particularly in the feet.

Note   Many patients with known diabetes, whether receiving treatmen or not, have no symptoms or signs of diabetes or its complications.

IV. Diagnostic studies

 A. Suggestive findings

  1. Glucose in the urine.

  2. Elevated glucose concentration in the blood. (This finding must be considered in relation to when the patient last ate.)

3. Acetone or blood in the urine. (This is generally seen when diabetes is out of control or when the patient, diabetic or not, is fasting.)

B. **Approach to diagnosis** There is now strong evidence suggesting that the metabolic component of diabetes with its high blood glucose level may not be causally related to the vascular component of diabetes, with its problems with the eyes, kidneys, nerves, and circulatory system. Therefore, there is little reason to justify aggressive diagnosis of asymptomatic diabetes. Glucose tolerance tests should be done only when it is important to make the diagnosis of diabetes, as in the patient with unexplained nervous system disease or hypoglycemic episodes. In general, a blood glucose drawn 2 hours after giving 100 gm of glucose is sufficient to make the diagnosis. All abnormal blood glucose levels in an undiagnosed patient should lead to a consultation with a physician.

V. Differential diagnosis

A. Diabetes mellitus must be differentiated from other causes of hyperglycemia:

1. Chronic pancreatitis (usually secondary to alcoholism).

2. Cushing's syndrome.

3. Drugs

a. Corticosteroids.

b. Diuretics.

B. Rarely, the renal threshold for glucose may be low and urine may be positive for glucose at a normal blood level. This is known as *renal glycosuria.*

VI. Treatment

A. General considerations before treating hyperglycemia

1. Precipitating factors should be looked for when diabetes is suddenly manifested or goes out of control in a previously stable patient. Factors to look for are:

a. Infection.

b. Pregnancy.

c. Drugs, such as thiazide diuretics or corticosteroids.

2. Treatment of blood glucose should be directed at keeping the

patient asymptomatic by lowering the blood sugar sufficiently to prevent polyuria and resultant dehydration and to prevent acidosis. Careful control of blood glucose does not retard vascular complications.

3. Closer control must be maintained in those patients who are prone to development of ketosis and thus subject to ketoacidosis These include almost all juvenile diabetics.

4. Although the vascular disease of diabetes cannot be prevented, as far as is known at the present time, careful skin hygiene and diligent foot care may prevent the development of dangerous complications, such as gangrene and amputation.

B. Treatment of the new diabetic

1. Evaluation

   a. Eye examination, with testing of visual acuity and funduscop:

   b. Examination of peripheral vascular system.

   c. Examination of nervous system.

   d. Urinalysis, with determination of BUN and creatinine levels.

   e. Electrocardiograph and chest x-ray.

   f. Cholesterol and triglyceride levels.

2. **Diet**   Obesity is a major predisposing factor to diabetes and all patients should attain normal weight. A diabetic reducing diet should be used until normal weight is attained and a maintenanc diet developed. Restriction of calories is more important than restriction of carbohydrates or other specific nutrients.

3. **Urine testing**

   a. The patient should be instructed on the proper method of collecting and testing urine and asked to keep a chart of glyco uria.

   b. Initially, urine should be tested 3 or 4 times a day.

   c. Thereafter, as his condition stabilizes, the patient may test urine once or twice a day.

   d. In follow-up, urine glucose values under 4+ will be sufficient judge the patient's control, and therapy may be maintained o basis of urine glucose levels alone. See Table 12-1 for comparison of sensitivity of different urine tests to glycosuria.

Table 12-1 Comparison of Urine Tests by "Percent"[a]

	0%	1/2%	1%	2%	3%	4%	5%
Clinitest two-drop method	N T 1+		2+	3+	4+		5+
Clinitest five-drop method	N T 1+ 2+		3+	4+			
Diastix	N T 1+ 2+		3+	4+			
Benedict's	N 1+		2+ 3+	4+			
TesTape	N 1+ 2+ 3+			4+			
Clinistix	N	*Light* means 1/4% or less; *dark* means 1/2% or more; *medium* means between 1/4% and 1/2%					

[a]*Percent (%)* = gm/100 ml; *N* = normal; *T* = trace.

4. **Instruction in personal hygiene**, especially foot care.

5. **Drug therapy**

   Note All diabetic therapy is based on patient education. To a degree not found in any other disease, the patient manages his own therapy. Good control and maintenance require the patient to observe his diet and test urine at home. All manipulation of medicines is useless in the face of an uncooperative or uneducated patient.

   a. If blood glucose concentration is less than 300 mg per 100 ml and the patient has no symptoms and no ketosis, institute patient education and diet.

   b. If blood glucose concentration is greater than 300 mg per 100 ml, consult physician about starting oral agents or insulin. Because a recent large study[*] indicated that tolbutamide may be related to increased mortality from arteriosclerotic heart disease, some physicians may choose to eliminate oral agents entirely or use them only after a consent form has been signed.

      (1) **Oral agents** Slowly (weekly or biweekly) increase dose until symptoms are relieved or the maximum dose is reached.

         (a) Tolbutamide (Orinase): Start with 500 or 1000 mg

[*]The University Group Diabetes Program. A study of the effects of hypoglycemic agents on vascular complications in patients with adult-onset diabetes. *Diabetes* 19(Suppl. 2): 747–830, 1970.

per day, given 2 or 3 times a day. Maximum dose is 2000 mg.

or

(b)   Chlorpropamide (Diabinese): Start with 250 mg per day, given once a day. Maximum dose is 750 mg.

(c)   Side-effects of oral agents

(1)   Hypoglycemia (more common in elderly patients on chlorpropamide).

(2)   Gastrointestinal disturbances.

(2)   Insulin   An initial dose must be decided on the basis of the patient's condition. The following are guidelines for the care of a patient newly started on insulin:

(a)   Instruct patient on the relation of insulin to blood glucose level, and time of peak effect of insulin:

(1)   Regular insulin: Peak effect 3—4 hours after injection.

(2)   Insulin lente (extended insulin zinc suspensi and NPH insulin (isophane insulin suspensio Peak effect 8—10 hours after injection.

(b)   Inform patient of the symptoms and treatment of hypoglycemia. **Note** Hypoglycemia itself causes primarily central nervous system disturbances; the symptoms of anxiety, sweating, and tachycardia are caused by epinephrine. Thus, confusion, abno mal behavior, or stupor may be the only signs of hypoglycemia.

(c)   Administration of insulin

(1)   Instruct patient in the care of needles and syringes (disposable ones are best).

(2)   Outline injection sites.

(3)   Observe patient drawing up insulin and self-administering it.

(d)   Test a fasting blood glucose specimen on the morn ing of the first injection.

    (e) Administer insulin. (This is a good time to instruct patient on insulin therapy and self-administration of insulin.)

    (f) Test a blood glucose specimen at 4—5 P.M. to check peak effect of insulin.

    (g) Give patient a chart for recording glycosuria. Check initially at 7 A.M., 11 A.M., 4 P.M., and 9 P.M. If this is too frequent for patient cooperation, 7 A.M. and 4 P.M. will suffice.

    (h) Schedule return visits at least once a week until diabetes is stable.

    (i) Increase insulin only in small increments, 3—4 units at a time. Blood glucose should be evaluated each time insulin dose is changed.

C. Maintenance

1. See patient regularly, depending on adequacy of control and level of complications.

2. Evaluate fasting blood glucose on each visit until control is achieved, then monitor with urine testing. Once the renal threshold is established, urine glucose levels below 4+ should be sufficient information.

3. Continue regular home monitoring of urine sugar.

4. Provide constant reminders of the necessity for dietary control, with careful attention to weight. (Weight loss may mean poor control of diabetes as well as good diet.)

5. Take an ECG every 5 years in premenopausal females, and every year in all other patients over age 30.

6. Carry out urinalysis and determination of the creatinine concentration every year.

7. Perform careful funduscopic, peripheral vascular, and neurologic examinations every year.

VII. Complications

A. Vascular complications.

B. Elevated blood glucose level with resultant polyuria.

C. Ketoacidosis in uncontrolled diabetes.

D. Tendency of infections to be more difficult to control and to occur more frequently.

E. Development of arteriosclerotic heart disease and peripheral vascular disease at an earlier age than nondiabetic persons.

VIII. **Consultation – referral**

A. All new diabetics.

B. Blood glucose concentration greater than 400 mg per 100 ml.

C. Refractory diabetes.

IX. **Follow-up**   See **VI.C.**

GOUT AND HYPERURICEMIA (Adult)

I. **Definition**   Gout is the result of an inborn error of metabolism leading to hyperuricemia that may be associated with acute inflammatory arthritis or monosodium urate deposits that appear as tophi. Only 10–20% of patients with clinically apparent gout give a positive family history.

II. **Etiology**

A. Primary gout is the result of an inborn error of metabolism.

B. Secondary hyperuricemia with or without symptoms of arthritis is associated with:

1. Drugs, e.g., thiazide diuretics.

2. Myeloproliferative diseases.

3. Chronic renal disease.

4. Obesity.

5. Starvation.

III. **Clinical features**

A. **Acute gout**

1. **Symptoms**

a. Painful, swollen joint.

b. Generally no systemic symptoms other than moderately elevated temperature in some cases.

2. Signs

   a. Red, hot, tender joint, with inflammation extending into the surrounding tissue.

   b. Usually, involvement of only one joint, with a strong predilection for the joints of the feet and ankles. Classically, gout appears in the big toe (podagra). Hips, shoulders, and vertebrae are rarely the site of gouty arthritis.

B. Chronic gout

   1. **Symptoms** The patient may be entirely asymptomatic between acute attacks of acute gout.

   2. **Signs**

      a. An elevated serum uric acid level (greater than 7.5 mg per 100 ml) may be the only manifestation. With treatment, the uric acid level may fall to normal.

      b. Uric acid deposits (tophi) are found in only a small number of patients having an initial clinical attack of gout. Thereafter, with recurrence, the incidence of tophi increases. Tophi characteristically are found in and around joints, bursae, and subcutareous tissue, especially around the olecranal bursa, the joints of the hand and foot, and the helix and anthelix of the ear.

      c. Kidney stones appear in about 40% of gouty patients with an elevated serum uric acid level.

IV. **Laboratory studies**

A. **Acute gout**

   1. Usually, the serum uric acid level is greater than 7.5 mg per 100 ml.

   2. Clinically affected joints contain urate crystals.

   3. White blood cell count usually is greater than 10,000 per cubic millimeter.

   4. Erythrocyte sedimentation rate may be elevated.

B. **Chronic gout**

   1. Serum uric acid level may be below normal, normal, or elevated.

   2. Erythrocyte sedimentation rate is normal.

   3. White blood cell count is normal.

V. **Differential diagnosis**   Acute gout.

A. Acute inflammatory monarthritis

1. Rheumatoid arthritis.

2. Pyogenic arthritis.

3. Pseudogout (chondrocalcinosis secondary to deposits of calcium pyrophosphate).

4. Reiter's disease.

5. Sarcoidosis.

B. Degenerative arthritis or osteoarthritis.

VI. **Treatment**

A. **Description of drugs**   Several drugs used in the treatment of gout have specific but different effects and must be used accordingly.

1. **Probenecid** (Benemid) blocks the reabsorption of uric acid by the proximal renal tubule. Probenecid, by causing increased excretion of uric acid, lowers the serum uric acid level. This drug is not of benefit in acute gout, but is used in maintenance of normal uric acid levels.

2. **Allopurinol** (Zyloprim) blocks the production of uric acid and thus decreases the serum uric acid level. This drug is used in maintenance therapy and is contraindicated in acute gout.

3. **Colchicine** has been used for many years **for acute attacks** of gouty arthritis. Colchicine's specific effect in terminating an acute attack of gout has diagnostic significance. Rarely is it used in maintenance therapy, the exception being in patients with chronic gout who have frequent acute attacks. In this situation it may reduce the frequency and severity of attacks.

4. **Indomethacin** (Indocin) and **phenylbutazone** (Butazolidin) are nonspecific antiinflammatory drugs that frequently **provide relief in acute gout.**

B. **Acute gout**

1. Colchicine, 1 mg initially, then 0.5 mg every hour until symptoms are relieved or diarrhea begins. No more than 6 mg should be given for any attack or over a 72-hour period.

   or

2. Indomethacin, 25 mg 3 times a day, is often effective and not associated with diarrhea.

   or

3. Phenylbutazone, 0.4–0.6 gm initially, then 0.2 gm every 4 hours to a total dose of 1 gm on days 1 and 2, then 0.1 gm 4 times a day for several days, then stop.

C. **Chronic gout**

   1. Known gout requires maintenance therapy with either:

      a. Probenecid, 500 mg twice a day, adjusted to serum uric acid level

         or

      b. Allopurinol, 100 mg 3 times a day, or a single 300-mg tablet given at 9 A.M.

   2. Which drug to use is still a matter of debate, but in patients with known gout and normal renal function, **probenecid is probably the drug of choice.** When therapy is initiated with either drug it may precipitate acute symptomatic gout (for unexplained reasons). The initial dose should be lower than the maintenance dose and should be given in conjunction with colchicine, 0.5 mg 4 times a day, for 1–2 weeks. Colchicine then may be discontinued and a maintenance dose begun that may have to be continued for life in order to keep the serum uric acid level between 6 and 7 mg per 100 ml.

D. Elevated uric acid level unassociated with symptoms of acute gout or any other evidence of uric acid elevation

   1. Less than 10 mg per 100 ml – no therapy.

   2. Greater than 10 mg per 100 ml on two successive occasions – allopurinol or probenecid may be used to lower serum uric acid level.

VII. **Complications**

A. Recurrent acute attacks without proper maintenance therapy can lead to chronic joint disability.

B. Untreated elevated serum uric acid level can result in the following:

   1. Acute gout.

    2. Renal stones with secondary infections or renal colic, or both.

    3. Tophaceous deposits in skin, joints, connective tissue.

VIII. Consultation — referral

A. New patient with acute gouty arthritis.

B. Patient known to have gouty arthritis who has frequent attacks.

C. Acute attack that persists beyond 72 hours.

IX. Follow-up

A. **Chronic gout** In asymptomatic chronic gout, uric acid levels need to be checked only twice a year.

B. **Acute gout** The patient should be telephoned or seen in 24 hours. A new patient should return in 1 week to begin maintenance therap

HYPOTHYROIDISM — MAINTENANCE OF DIAGNOSED DISEASE (Adult)

I. **Definition** Decreased function of the thyroid gland, causing a reduced production of thyroid hormone and leading to progressive slowing of a bodily functions.

II. **Etiology** Hypothyroidism is caused by thyroid failure due to a numbe of mechanisms:

A. Treatment of hyperthyroidism (radioiodine, surgery, propylthiourac

B. Following thyroiditis.

C. Idiopathic thyroid failure.

D. Congenital defects in thyroid metabolism.

E. Rarely, iodine insufficiency.

III. **Clinical features** The adequately treated patient should be euthyroid, without signs of hyperthyroidism or hypothyroidism:

A. **Hypothyroidism**

    1. **Symptoms**

        a. Decreased energy, lethargy.

        b. Cold intolerance.

        c. Constipation.

      d. Menorrhagia.

      e. Sometimes, slight weight gain late in disease.

  2. **Signs**

      a. Dry hair, which may fall out.

      b. Dry, rough skin.

      c. Hoarseness.

      d. Periorbital edema, dull expression.

      e. Slow Achilles tendon reflex (return phase).

B. Hyperthyroidism (Graves' disease)

  1. **Symptoms**

      a. Nervousness.

      b. Heat intolerance.

      c. Weight loss.

      d. Increased appetite.

      e. Increased sweating.

      f. Emotional instability.

  2. **Signs**

      a. Sweating; moist skin.

      b. Tachycardia.

      c. Arrhythmia (primarily in older age group).

      d. Fine tremor of fingers ("cat's purr") and tongue.

      e. Lid lag.

IV. Laboratory studies

  A. Euthyroidism: The values of protein-bound iodine (PBI), serum triiodothyronine (T_3) uptake, and serum thyroxine (T_4) using the Murphy-Pattee method are normal if the patient is taking desiccated thyroid. PBI and T_4 are low if the patient is taking sodium liothyronine (Cytomel).

  B. Hypothyroidism: Decreased PBI, T_3 uptake, and T_4.

  C. Hyperthyroidism: Increased PBI, T_3 uptake, and T_4.

Note   Birth control pills increase PBI and decrease T_3 uptake because of increased protein substrate for binding. All iodine-containing medicines and x-ray procedures using iodine-containing media will contaminate PBI, giving falsely high values (usually extremely high and obviously secondary to contamination). For these reasons the Murphy-Pattee technique for determining T_4, if available, is the most accurate and reliable test.

V. **Differential diagnosis**   If laboratory data do not reveal any evidence of thyroid dysfunction, one must find other causes of the symptoms and clinical findings.

VI. **Treatment**

A. Continue replacement therapy, adjusting according to clinical response and PBI and T_4 results.

B. Usual doses of thyroid replacement

1. Thyroid extract, 1½–2½ grains (100–200 mg) orally every day.

2. Sodium levothyroxine (Synthroid), 0.1 mg orally 2 or 3 times a day.

3. Sodium liothyronine (Cytomel), 25–75 μg orally every day.

VII. **Complications**

A. Hypothyroidism.

B. Hyperthyroidism.

VIII. **Consultation – referral**   Development of hyperthyroid signs and symptoms.

IX. **Follow-up**   Test for PBI or T_4 approximately once a year or when patient's condition changes.

MULTINODULAR GOITER (Adult)

I. **Definition**   Enlargement of the thyroid in which there is more than one identifiable nodule, occurring in females 10 to 20 times more frequently than in males.

II. **Etiology**   Unknown. An inborn metabolic block may be responsible. Rarely is this disorder secondary to iodine deficiency in the United States today.

III. Clinical features

A. Symptoms

1. Generally patients are euthyroid, although occasionally after many years symptoms of hyperthyroidism may develop.

2. Symptoms of tracheal compression (stridor, difficult breathing) may develop if enlargement is great.

B. Signs

1. Visible swelling of neck.

2. Palpable thyroid with more than one nodule.

3. Nonpulsatile, nontender mass.

IV. Laboratory studies Generally, results of thyroid studies are normal, except in the rare case of hyperthyroid goiter. Measurement of serum thyroxine (T_4) by the Murphy-Pattee method should be carried out.

V. Differential diagnosis

A. Solitary thyroid nodule.

B. Hashimoto's thyroiditis.

VI. Treatment

A. If the patient is euthyroid, treatment is not indicated unless the gland is cosmetically disfiguring or causing obstruction. In these cases thyroid extract, 1–2 grains daily, may be used for suppressing the pituitary and reducing the size of the thyroid gland.

B. Significant compression may require surgery.

VII. Complications

A. Hyperthyroidism.

B. Tracheal obstruction.

C. Rarely, thyroid carcinoma in an enlarged gland.

VIII. Consultation – referral

A. Obstructive symptoms.

B. Hyperthyroidism.

C. Solitary nodule.

D. Goiter in males, especially young males.

E. A tender thyroid gland.

IX. Follow-up

A. Every 6 months if gland is medically treated.

B. Every year if untreated.

IRON DEFICIENCY ANEMIA (Pediatric)

I. **Definition**

  A. **Anemia** in general may be defined on the basis of a lowered hematocrit reading.

Age	Hematocrit (%)
3–6 months	Less than 30
6 months–6 years	Less than 33
6–14 years	Less than 34
Over 14 years	
Female	Less than 36
Male	Less than 40

  B. **Iron deficiency anemia** is a form of anemia resulting from an inadequate supply of iron for synthesis of hemoglobin.

II. **Etiology** More than one of the following factors may be causative in an individual patient:

  A. Inadequate supply of iron at birth

    1. Prematurity.

    2. Fetal or perinatal blood loss without replacement.

  B. Inadequate dietary iron.

  C. Excessive demands for iron associated with growth

    1. Prematurely born infant.

    2. Adolescent.

  D. Blood loss without replacement

    1. Blood loss may be obvious.

    2. The most common occult source of blood loss is the gastrointestinal tract.

III. Clinical features

A. History   One or more of the following factors may be relevant:

1. Premature birth without supplemental iron or iron-fortified milk during first year of life. Such an infant will usually be anemic by age 9 months on an average diet.

2. Iron-deficient diet. When milk not fortified with iron accounts for a large proportion of an infant's caloric intake, the overall diet will probably be poor in iron because of the low iron content of milk. Anemia from this cause is most common between 9 and 24 months of age. During the adolescent growth period, the incidence of iron deficiency anemia from an iron-deficient diet increases again, especially in females.

3. Large intake of whole cow's milk during first two years of life. This may be associated with gastrointestinal blood loss as well as a diet poor in iron.

4. Blood loss without replacement.

B. Symptoms

1. Mild iron deficiency anemia (hematocrit reading 25–33%)

   a. This is usually asymptomatic and discovered during routine health maintenance screening.

   b. Results of some studies have suggested the possibility that decreased attention span may be associated with iron deficiency even before anemia develops.

2. More severe iron deficiency anemia (hematocrit reading less than 25%)

   a. Pallor.

   b. Lethargy.

   c. Irritability.

   d. Anorexia.

   e. Occasionally, poor weight gain.

C. Signs

1. Mild iron deficiency anemia: Normal physical examination.

2. More severe iron deficiency anemia

  a. Pallor.

  b. Occasional findings

     (1) Poor weight gain.

     (2) Splenomegaly.

     (3) Systolic flow murmurs.

IV. Laboratory studies

A. Hematocrit An abnormal value requires a repeat determination.

B. Smear of red blood cells for morphology If anemia is more than mild, the red blood cells are hypochromic and microcytic, with some variety of size and shape.

V. Differential diagnosis

A. Anemia in general

1. Acute or chronic hemorrhage.

2. Excessive red blood cell destruction, as in hemolytic anemias such as sickle cell anemia and other hereditary anemias.

3. Decreased or impaired production of red blood cells, as in iron deficiency anemia, chronic infection, renal failure, and leukemia.

B. Iron deficiency anemia One should try to establish why the patient is iron deficient (see **II** and **III.A**).

VI. Treatment

A. Indications for treatment without consultation Treatment for iron deficiency anemia may be started without consultation and before results of red blood cell smear are known if all of the following circumstances apply:

1. Hematocrit reading greater than 24% but less than normal.

2. Patient more than 10 months of age.

3. No history of a normal hematocrit or hemoglobin value in the past.

4. No history of unexplained blood loss, e.g., red blood in stools or tarry stools.

5. No history in siblings of anemia due to a cause other than iron deficiency.

6. No abnormality on physical examination not explained by an unrelated diagnosis.

B. **Therapeutic measures**

1. **Discontinue whole cow's milk in infant** under 18 months, substituting evaporated milk formula or commercial infant formula.

2. **Decrease total milk intake** to no more than 16 ounces a day and **increase other foods**, especially those with high iron content, e.g. egg yolk, liver, turkey, red meat, bran flakes, dried fruit (raisins, prunes, peaches, apricots), and beans (red kidney, pinto, lima).

3. **Iron therapy**　6—7 mg per kilogram of body weight (3 mg per pound) of elemental iron per day in three divided doses for 2 months (see Table 13-1).

C. **Prevention**

1. **Full-term infant**

   a. Iron-fortified milk until age 18 months

   or

   b. Medicinal iron supplement from 3—18 months of age (see Table 13-2 for dosage) unless baby consumes a solid diet high in iron content (see **VI.B.2**).

   c. Intake of iron-containing foods.

Table 13-1　Oral Dosage of Ferrous Sulfate (Fer-In-Sol) for Treatment of Iron Deficiency Anemia

Drug Form	Body Weight	Dose	Frequency
Ferrous sulfate drops (15 mg elemental iron per 0.6 ml)	8—10 kg (18—22 lb) 10—12 kg (22—26 lb)	0.6 ml[a] 0.9 ml[a]	3 times a day aft meals for 2 mo
or			
Ferrous sulfate syrup (6 mg elemental iron per milliliter)	12—16 kg (26—35 lb) 16—22 kg (35—48 lb) 22—30 kg (48—66 lb)	5.0 ml 7.5 ml 10.0 ml	3 times a day aft meals for 2 mo
or			
Ferrous sulfate capsules (60 mg elemental iron per capsule)	Over 30 kg (over 66 lb)	1 capsule	3 times a day aft meals for 2 mo

[a]May be given in water, fruit juice, or vegetable juice.

Table 13-2   Oral Pediatric Dosage of Ferrous Sulfate Drops (Fer-In-Sol) (15 mg elemental iron per 0.6 ml)

Body Weight	Dose[a]	Frequency
4–7 kg (9–15 lb)	0.3 ml	Once a day
Over 7 kg (over 15 lb)	0.6 ml	Once a day until age 18 months

[a]May be given in water, fruit juice, or vegetable juice.

2. **Premature infant**

   a. Iron-fortified milk until age 18 months

     or

   b. Medicinal iron supplement from 2–18 months of age: ferrous sulfate drops (Fer-In-Sol) (containing 15 mg elemental iron per 0.6 ml) in a dosage of 0.6 ml. once a day in water, fruit juice, or vegetable juice.

   c. Intake of iron-containing foods.

VII. **Complications**

  A. Progressive anemia, with increasing symptoms.

  B. Accidental ingestion of medicinal iron, especially capsules, resulting in fatal iron intoxication. Like all medications it should be locked away from young children.

VIII. **Consultation – referral**

  A. Hematocrit reading less than 25%.

  B. Patient less than 10 months of age.

  C. History of a normal hematocrit or hemoglobin in the past.

  D. History of unexplained blood loss, e.g., red blood in stools or tarry stools.

  E. History in siblings of anemia due to a cause other than iron deficiency.

  F. Abnormality on physical examination not explained by an unrelated diagnosis.

  G. Abnormal red blood cell morphology.

  H. Failure of hematocrit to return to normal in 1 month despite iron therapy.

IX. **Follow-up**

  A. Clinic visit after 1 month of iron therapy

   1. Determination of hematocrit reading (should be normal).

   2. Review of diet and further counseling as needed.

  B. Clinic visit after 2 months of iron therapy

   1. Determination of hematocrit reading (should remain at or above 1-month level).

   2. Review of diet and further counseling as needed.

  C. Clinic visit 9 months after discontinuing iron therapy

   1. Determination of hematocrit reading (should remain normal).

   2. Review of diet and further counseling as needed.

IRON DEFICIENCY ANEMIA IN MENSTRUATING FEMALE

  I. **Definition**   Hematocrit reading less than 38% in menstruating females. The anemia is usually secondary to chronic iron loss and may be aggravated by the intake of a diet low in iron as a result of food faddism or socioeconomic factors.

 II. **Etiology**   See **I.**

III. **Clinical features**

  A. **Symptoms**

   1. There may be none and anemia may be discovered on routine blood examination.

   2. Fatigue, weakness, headache, dizziness, and other nonspecific generalized complaints may be present but are very nonspecific.

  B. **Signs**

   1. Sometimes, none.

   2. Pallor of skin and conjunctiva.

   3. Fissure of lips.

   4. Brittle nails.

   5. Sometimes, heavy menstrual periods.

IV. **Laboratory studies**

  A. **Studies required before treatment**

    1. Complete blood count, hematocrit determination, white blood cell count, differential count, and red cell indices.

    2. Stool benzidine test (on three separate specimens if possible).

    3. Sickledex test if patient is a black person.

  B. **Findings in optional studies**

    1. Microcytic and hypochromic red blood cells are seen on smear.

    2. Mean corpuscular hemoglobin is less than 27 $\mu\mu$g; mean corpuscular volume is less than 83 μ^3.

    3. Serum iron saturation is less than 20%; serum iron-binding capacity is greater than normal.

V. **Differential diagnosis**

  A. **Iron deficiency anemia secondary to menstruation** must be differentiated from other causes of iron loss, which are usually from the gastrointestinal tract. Thus, results of stool benzidine test must be negative.

  B. **Anemia secondary to ineffective production**

    1. Bone marrow depression from drugs, infections, lead poisoning.

    2. Defective hemoglobin (e.g., sickle cell).

    3. Vitamin deficiency (B_{12}, folic acid).

    4. Chronic disease.

  C. **Anemia from hemolysis.**

VI. **Treatment**   Ferrous sulfate, 300 mg orally three times a day for 3 months.

VII. **Complications**   Rare.

VIII. **Consultation – referral**

  A. Menstruating female with hematocrit reading less than 30%.

  B. Menstruating female with positive stool benzidine test results.

  C. Failure to improve after 1 month of treatment.

  D. All other cases of anemia.

    E. Patients in whom serum iron or red blood cell indices, or both, do not fit iron deficiency anemia.

IX. Follow-up   Repeat hematocrit determination in 1 month.

Obstetrics and Gynecology

GUIDELINES FOR MANAGING THE OBSTETRIC PATIENT

I. **Prenatal care**   All data should be recorded on the prenatal record (Fig. 14-1).

A. **The first visit**

1. **Examination**   The first examination should be done by the family nurse practitioner (FNP), preferably after the second missed period, unless the patient is having some trouble, such as severe nausea, vomiting, pain, or bleeding.

   a. A complete history and physical examination should be performed.

   b. The pelvic examination should include obtaining a Papanicolaou smear and gonococcal culture from the cervix.

   c. The initial pregnancy laboratory work should include the following studies or determinations:

      (1)   Serology.

      (2)   Blood type and Rh factor.

      (3)   Antibody screening.

      (4)   Rubella titer.

      (5)   Hematocrit.

      (6)   Urinalysis.

2. **Medications**

   a. A routine prenatal vitamin with folic acid should be started at this time.

   b. Ferrous sulfate, 300 mg 3 times a day, should also be started if the hematocrit reading is below 36%.

3. **Patient instruction**

   a. The FNP should instruct the patient concerning diet and personal hygiene.

Name _____

Race _____ Marital status _____ Age _____ Years married _____ Years education _____ Religion _____ Occupation _____
 S.M.W.D. Sep.

Father of child

Name _____ Birthplace _____ Age _____

Occupation _____ Business address or employer _____

Significant diseases _____ Height _____ Weight _____ Blood group _____ Rh _____

Previous obstetric history

Full-term _____ Premature _____ Abortions _____ Alive _____

No.	Year	Place of Confinement	Weeks of Gestation	Type of Delivery	Duration of Labor	Compli-cations	Apgar I	Condition at Birth	Child Weight	Present Condition	Icterus	Rh Type	Anal-gesia	Anes-thesia
1														
2														
3														
4														
5														
6														
7														
8														
9														
10														

Figure 14-1 Obstetric prenatal record sheet.

Eclampsia _____	Edema _____	Hyperemesis _____
Toxemia _____	Urinary tract infection _____	Rh difficulty _____
Lactation difficulty _____		

Family history (tuberculosis, hypertension, heart disease, diabetes, neuropsychiatric disorders, epilepsy, allergies, multiple births, congenital anomalies)

_____

Medical history

Blood transfusion _____	Diabetes _____	Allergy _____
Bleeding tendency _____	Hepatitis or jaundice _____	Thyroid _____
Hypertension _____	Nephritis _____	Venereal disease _____
Heart disease _____	Pyelitis, cystitis _____	Anemia _____
Phlebitis _____	Tuberculosis _____	German measles _____

Infertility _____

Operations and accidents _____

General health _____

Menstrual history

Onset at _____ years. Interval _____ days. Duration _____ days.

Irregularities _____ Dysmenorrhea _____

Coital difficulties _____

Figure 14-1 *(Continued)*

Present pregnancy

Date: Last menstruation _____ Quickening _____

Expected date of
confinement: From data _____ From examination _____

Contraceptive used _____ When discontinued _____ Pregnancy planned _____

Headache _____ Vomiting _____ Indigestion _____ Constipation _____

Nausea _____ Edema _____ Vision _____ Backache _____

Leukorrhea _____ Bleeding _____ Pelvic pain _____

Height _____ Usual weight _____ Present weight _____

Remarks _____

Initial physical examination

Date _____

T. ___ P. ___ R. ___ B.P. ___ General nutrition _____

Oral cavity _____ Eyes _____ Optic fundi _____

Breasts _____ Nipples _____ Thyroid _____

Heart _____

Lungs _____

Kidney, liver, spleen _____

Abdominal scars _____ Height of fundus _____ Fetal heartbeat _____

Est. fetal weight _____ Presentation and position _____ Duration of pregnancy _____

Orthopedic defects _____ Varicosities _____ Edema _____

Figure 14-1 *(Continued)*

Initial pelvic examination

Outlet _____

Cervix _____

Uterus _____

Adnexa _____

Discharge _____ Rectal examination _____

Pelvic measurements

Examined by Dr. _____

C. D. _____ T. I. _____ Arch. _____ C. D. _____ T. I. _____ Arch. _____
P. S. _____

Sacrum _____ Coccyx _____ Sacrum _____ Coccyx _____

Sidewalls _____ Spines _____ SS Lig _____ SS Notch _____

_____

X-ray pelvimetry

Date _____ Morphology _____

Trans. inlet _____ I. S. _____ T. I. _____

O. C. _____ P. S. M. _____ P. S. O. _____

Read by _____ A. P. M. _____ A. P. O. _____

Figure 14-1 *(Continued)*

Results of examination							Estimated date of confinement				
Date											
Duration of gestation											
Vomiting											
Headaches											
Constipation											
Bleeding											
Upper respiratory infection											
Rash, fever											
Emotional problems											
Weight (normal)											
Weight gain/Total											
Edema											
Blood pressure											
Urine albumin/sugar											
Hemoglobin Hematocrit											
Fetal position											
Fetal heartbeat											
Height of fundus											
Fetal weight											
Medications Immunizations											
Examiner											

Figure 14-1 *(Continued)*

Blood group _____ Rh _____ STS _____ Prenatal vitamin _____ Date _____

Type _____ Date _____ Prenatal iron _____ Date _____

Anti-Rh titer _____

Parents' classes _____

Physical therapy _____

Type _____ Date _____

X-rays _____ Analgesia preference _____

_____ Anesthesia preference _____

_____ Nursing preference _____

Figure 14-1 *(Continued)*

    b. The patient should be told to report to the FNP any of the following conditions:

       (1) Persistent vomiting.

       (2) Continuous or severe headaches.

       (3) Persistent or recurring abdominal pain.

       (4) Vaginal bleeding.

       (5) Dimness or blurring of vision.

       (6) Chills or fever.

       (7) Loss of fluid from vagina (not vaginal discharge, but a gush of watery-type fluid or a continuous loss of this fluid).

       (8) Swelling of hands, feet, or face that becomes persistent.

       (9) Urinary symptoms, e.g., dysuria or hematuria.

B. The second visit

1. The second visit is made *4 weeks later.*

2. Examination is done together by the obstetrician and the FNP.

3. The obstetrician should confirm the diagnosis of pregnancy and measure the pelvis.

C. Subsequent visits

1. **Scheduling**　Unless some special instructions are given by the obstetrician, the subsequent prenatal examinations should be done by the FNP at the following intervals:

    a. Every 4 weeks until 28 weeks of gestation.

    b. Every 2 weeks from 28–36 weeks of gestation.

    c. Every week from 36 weeks until delivery.

2. **Routine studies**

    a. Every routine prenatal examination should include:

       (1) Questioning the patient about any present problems.

       (2) Blood pressure.

       (3) Urinalysis.

        (4)   Measurement of the uterine fundus.

        (5)   Auscultation of the fetal heart.

        (6)   Determination of the position of the fetus, if possible.

   b. Hematocrit determination should be repeated at 24 and 34 weeks in each patient, and at every visit with a reading below 36%.

3. Examination   If possible, prenatal examinations should be done by the FNP on the same day the obstetrician is to be at the clinic, but before he arrives, so that any problem case may be held over for him to see.

4. Assessment of Rh-negative patients   At the initial prenatal screening examination, blood is drawn for blood type and Rh factor determination. All Rh-negative patients are to be handled as follows:

   a. Antibody titer is measured when the patient is discovered to be Rh-negative.

   b. Rh antibody titer determination is repeated in Rh-negative patients at 24 and 34 weeks of gestation.

   c. Patients found to have a *positive* Rh antibody titer, either initially or on repeat studies, should be referred to the obstetrician.

   d. Patients who are *Rh negative, D^u positive,* are treated as if they were *Rh negative,* (i.e., there is no need for antibody titer determination or use of RhoGAM). Human Rh_0D immune globulin (RhoGAM) is given immediately after delivery to all unsensitized Rh-negative women to protect them against being sensitized in future pregnancies.

D. Referral

1. The FNP should consult with or refer the patient to the obstetrician if any of the following are noted:

   a. No fetal heart tones are heard by 22 weeks.

   b. The patient feels no movement by 22 weeks or none for 1 week at any time after this.

   c. Blood pressure is above 140/90 mm Hg on two checks after bedrest.

d. Patient has albuminuria or persistent edema.

e. Patient has glycosuria.

f. There is lack of regular fetal growth.

g. Late in pregnancy the FNP questions the position of the fetus, e.g., breech or transverse lie.

h. At any time that the FNP is in doubt about the patient's status.

i. Hematocrit reading is below 33%.

2. *All* prenatal patients should again be reviewed with and examined by the obstetrician at 36 weeks.

E. **General instruction relative to labor and delivery**   At some time, preferably between 28 and 32 weeks, but certainly before 36 weeks, the FNP should discuss with each patient when to go to the hospital:

1. **Contractions**

   a. Primigravidas should usually wait until contractions are regular at least 6–8 minutes apart, and lasting more then 30 seconds.

   b. Multigravidas probably should wait until the contractions are regular and 10–15 minutes apart.

   c. Instructions to patients, especially multigravidas, should be individualized according to the distance they must travel or history of previous rapid labor.

2. **Rupture of the membranes**   Patients should go directly to the hospital.

3. **Any active bleeding** (even without associated labor contractions): The patient should be instructed to go to the hospital. Discussion here should include differentiation of a small bloody mucous type of discharge from active bleeding. Explain to the patient that a bloody mucous discharge associated with contractions is a good sign that the contractions are true instead of false. A bloody mucous discharge by itself *without any contractions* may occur in the latter part of the pregnancy without indicating the immediate onset of labor.

4. **Onset of active labor**

   a. The patient should be instructed not to eat if she believes labor has started.

      b. She should be directed to report to the obstetrician at the hospital, who will then perform a vaginal examination to determine whether active labor has started. In most cases this is impossible to determine on the telephone by either the FNP or the physician. The decision whether the patient will be admitted in active labor or sent home if it is false labor will be made at the time of this examination.

    5. No *commitment* should be made by the FNP about the type of premedication in labor, the anesthetic for delivery, the physician who will perform the delivery, or the length of stay in the hospital. These will be determined at the time the patient is in active labor by the personnel at the hospital. The patient should understand the various types of anesthetics available and may have her preference noted on her obstetric record. Preference for breast- or bottle-feeding should also be recorded at this time. If there are any special questions about the foregoing, they may be discussed with the obstetrician when he sees the patient at 36 weeks.

II. Postpartum period

  A. Family planning The family nurse practitioner should discuss with the patient during pregnancy the type of birth control desired post partum:

    1. If the patient desires **oral contraceptives,** these may be started upon leaving the hospital. If they are not started then, the patient should telephone the FNP within the first two weeks after returning home to obtain the pills.

    2. If the patient desires an **intrauterine contraceptive device,** she should be brought in at 3 weeks post partum for insertion of the intrauterine contraceptive device by the physician.

    3. Candidates for **postpartum tubal sterilization** should be informed about the procedure and then evaluated by the obstetrician *before delivery.* Consent papers should be signed more than 30 days before delivery and attached to the hospital record.

    4. If the patient desires to use a **diaphragm,** she should return to the clinic 3 weeks post partum for fitting and instructions.

  B. Postpartum examinations

    1. All patients should be seen 4–6 weeks post partum for a **general physical examination, including breast and pelvic examination, plus laboratory work, including hematocrit determination and**

urinalysis. These examinations should be done by the obstetricia in association *with the FNP*.

2. **A Papanicolaou smear** should be done at this time if there is any question about the previous smear, or if for some reason a smear was not obtained during pregnancy.

NAUSEA AND VOMITING DURING PREGNANCY

I. **Definition**   Nausea and vomiting occurring alone or together during th course of pregnancy, usually during the first trimester.

II. **Etiology**   Unknown. Nausea and vomiting probably are related to the hormonal changes occurring with pregnancy, with psychologic factors playing a secondary but important role.

III. **Clinical features**

A. **Symptoms**

1. Nausea and vomiting, typically occurring early in the morning an then disappearing later in the day.

2. No abdominal pain or disturbance in bowel function.

B. **Signs**

1. No signs of dehydration.

2. Soft abdomen, with no tenderness. Normal bowel sounds.

IV. **Laboratory studies**   None.

V. **Differential diagnosis**

A. Hyperemesis gravidarum.

B. Viral gastroenteritis.

VI. **Treatment**

A. Frequent small feedings.

B. Bendectin (a combination of an antispasmodic, an antihistaminic, and vitamin B_6), 2 tablets orally at bedtime and then 1 or 2 tablets orally on arising.

VII. **Complications**   Dehydration.

VIII. **Consultation – referral**

A. Nausea or vomiting occurring later than twentieth week of pregnancy

    B. Dehydration.

    C. Persistence of nausea and vomiting that is annoying to patient even in the absence of dehydration.

IX. Follow-up

    A. Maintain daily contact for severe nausea and vomiting.

    B. Maintain weekly or less frequent contact if the problem is mild.

CANDIDAL VAGINITIS (Adult)

  I. Definition   An inflammatory process involving the vagina caused by a common skin fungus.

  II. Etiology   *Candida albicans.* Infection often occurs in association with uncontrolled diabetes mellitus, pregnancy, antibiotic usage, and use of birth control pills.

III. Clinical features

    A. Symptoms

        1. Vaginal discharge.

        2. Commonly, intense vulval itching or burning, or both.

        3. No vaginal bleeding.

    B. Signs

        1. Often, intense vulval inflammation.

        2. Copious cheesy vaginal discharge.

        3. Often, presence of cheesy discharge in labial folds.

        4. Sometimes, satellite lesions apart from the main area of inflammation.

IV. Laboratory studies

    A. Potassium hydroxide preparation is positive for *Candida.*

    B. Wet preparation is negative for *Trichomonas.*

    C. Urine should be tested for glycosuria.

    D. If there is a family history of diabetes or any symptoms suggestive of diabetes are present, or both, a blood glucose specimen is drawn 2 hours after eating.

V. **Differential diagnosis**

   A. Other causes of vaginitis.

   B. Carcinoma of the vagina or cervix, or both.

VI. **Treatment**

   A. If candidal vaginitis occurs in a patient with diabetes mellitus, the diabetes must be controlled before it is possible to control or cure the vaginitis.

   B. Nystatin (Mycostatin) vaginal tablets, 1 vaginally twice a day for 2 weeks, may be prescribed.

   C. Cool compresses may be applied to irritated vulval lesions twice a day. Dry the skin thoroughly before using a compress.

VII. **Complications** None.

VIII. **Consultation – referral**

   A. Refractory cases not responding to treatment in 2 weeks.

   B. Patient with coexisting uncontrolled or newly diagnosed diabetes.

IX. **Follow-up** As needed.

ABNORMAL PAPANICOLAOU SMEAR FINDINGS IN AN ASYMPTOMATIC PATIENT (Adult)

I. **Definition** A report on a cytologic examination of a cervical scraping taken from an *asymptomatic* patient that is read as abnormal, with abnormalities classified as follows:

   A. Inflammatory reaction (class II).

   B. Suggestive of malignancy, but not highly so (class III).

   C. Highly suggestive of malignancy (class IV).

   D. "Diagnostic" of malignancy (class V).

II. **Etiology**

   A. Many factors may lead to abnormal findings on a Papanicolaou smear, but **inflammation secondary to infections** is probably the most common cause.

   B. The possibility of a **malignancy** must always be considered.

III. **Clinical features**   Papanicolaou smears are most commonly done as a screening procedure and usually no complaints are present.

IV. **Laboratory studies**   None are indicated beyond the Papanicolaou smear itself and those studies indicated for vaginitis (see Candidal Vaginitis [Adult], **IV**, Trichomonal Vaginitis [Adult], **IV**, and Nonspecific or Bacterial Vaginitis [Adult], **IV**).

V. **Differential diagnosis**

   A. Malignancy.

   B. Inflammatory conditions.

   C. Laboratory error.

VI. **Treatment**

   A. For all class II findings, do a repeat smear in 6 months.

   B. For all class III findings, do a repeat smear in 4 weeks.

   C. If repeat smear is class III, IV, or V, refer patient.

   D. If repeat smear is normal (class I or II), do another repeat smear in 6 months.

   E. Treat nonspecific vaginitis, if present (see Nonspecific or Bacterial Vaginitis [Adult], **VI**).

   F. Do not treat trichomonads identified on Papanicolaou smear unless there are accompanying symptoms appropriate to *Trichomonas* infestation (see Trichomonal Vaginitis [Adult]).

VII. **Complications**   None.

VIII. **Consultation – referral**

   A. Smears highly suggestive of malignancy (class IV or V).

   B. Repeat smear that is again suggestive of malignancy (class III).

   C. The presence of any signs or symptoms suggestive of malignancy.

IX. **Follow-up**   See VI.

TRICHOMONAL VAGINITIS (Adult)

I. **Definition**   An inflammatory process involving the vagina caused by a common flagellate parasite.

II. **Etiology**　*Trichomonas.*

III. **Clinical features**

  A. **Symptoms**

    1. Vaginal discharge.

    2. Vulval itching.

    3. No vaginal bleeding.

  B. **Signs**

    1. Minimal vulval inflammation.

    2. Frothy, bubbly vaginal discharge.

IV. **Laboratory studies**

  A. Wet preparation is positive for *Trichomonas.*

  B. Potassium hydroxide preparation is negative for *Candida.*

V. **Differential diagnosis**　Other causes of vaginitis.

VI. **Treatment**

  A. **Nonpregnant patient**　Metronidazole (Flagyl) tablets, 1 orally 3 times a day for 10 days. Sexual partner should be treated also with Flagyl tablets, 1 orally twice a day for 10 days.

  B. **Pregnant patient**

    1. *Do not* use metronidazole.

    2. Use diiodohydroxyquin (Floraquin) vaginal suppositories, 2 vaginally at bedtime for 2 weeks.

Note:　Alcoholic beverages should not be taken during the course of Flagyl therapy.

VII. **Complications**　None.

VIII. **Consultation – referral**　Refractory cases not responding to treatment in 2 weeks.

IX. **Follow-up**　As needed.

NONSPECIFIC OR BACTERIAL VAGINITIS (Adult)

I. **Definition**　An inflammation of the vagina caused by one or more bacteria.

II. **Etiology**   Various bacteria.

III. **Clinical features**

   A. **Symptoms**

   1. Minimal vulval pruritus.

   2. Vaginal discharge.

   B. **Signs**   Yellowish white vaginal discharge.

IV. **Laboratory studies**

   A. Potassium hydroxide preparation is negative for *Candida.*

   B. Hanging-drop preparation is negative for *Trichomonas.*

   C. Culture for *Neisseria gonorrhoeae* is negative.

V. **Differential diagnosis**   Other causes of vaginitis, principally *Candida* and *Trichomonas.*

VI. **Treatment**

   A. Sultrin vaginal cream (a combination of sulfonamides), 1 applicatorful twice a day for 10 days

   or

   B. AVC vaginal cream (a combination of sulfanilamide and aminacrine HCl), 1 applicatorful twice a day for 10 days.

VII. **Complications**   None.

VIII. **Consultation – referral**   Refractory cases not responding to treatment in 2 weeks.

IX. **Follow-up**   As needed.

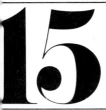

Parasitic Infestations

ASCARIASIS (Pediatric and Adult)

I. **Definition** Intestinal infestation by *Ascaris lumbricoides,* the human roundworm. It is seen most commonly in children, or in adults living with infested children.

II. **Etiology** *A. lumbricoides* become established in the gastrointestinal tract when eggs from soil or fecally contaminated fingers are ingested. Larvae migrate through the lungs and back to the small intestine, where they live unattached to the small intestine and grow to adult worms. The adult worm measures 16–35 cm in length by 2–6 mm in greatest diameter.

II. **Clinical features**

A. **Symptoms**

1. Many patients are asymptomatic.

2. Cough is produced during migration of the larvae through the lungs. Larvae may be coughed up and seen. Pulmonary syndrome may also include fever and pulmonary infiltrate.

3. Nausea, vomiting, anorexia, weight loss, and malaise occur with heavy infestation.

4. Children with pica are more likely to ingest eggs.

B. **Signs**

1. Larvae may be coughed up and identified.

2. Adult worms may be seen in the stool.

3. Failure to grow or weight loss may be present, especially in small children.

IV. **Laboratory studies**

A. None are needed if worms are seen.

B. Microscopic examination of stool may be done to detect eggs.

V. **Differential diagnosis**

    A. Other causes of failure to gain weight should be ruled out.

    B. Other causes of vague abdominal complaints should be ruled out.

    C. Pulmonary syndrome is often confused with bacterial or viral pneumonia or asthma.

    D. Ascariasis does not cause anemia, diarrhea, or malabsorption.

VI. **Treatment**

    A. Instruct family in **personal hygiene**, especially hand washing before eating and after using the toilet.

    B. Counsel parents on **prevention of pica**.

    C. **Specific therapy**   Treat all family members at the same time, using pyrantel pamoate (Antiminth) suspension given as a single oral dose of 1 ml per 5 kg (10 lb) of body weight. Maximum dose is 20 ml.

VII. **Complications**   Rarely, intestinal obstruction results from a tangled worm mass.

VIII. **Consultation – referral**   Generally not needed in routine cases.

IX. **Follow-up**   High-risk families with proved infection should be followed with periodic stool examinations because of the possibility of reinfection

PEDICULOSIS (Pediatric and Adult)

I. **Definition**   Infestation of the skin or hair by one or both of the two species of lice capable of infesting the human host.

II. **Etiology**

    A. *Pediculus humanis* infests the head or body.

    B. *Phthirus pubis,* the crab louse, infests the genital region.

    C. Both species of lice are transmitted either by close personal contact or through shared clothing, bedclothes, etc.

III. **Clinical features**

    A. **Symptoms**   Intense itching.

    B. **Signs**

        1. Head (pediculosis capitis)

    a. The nits (ova) are seen as small (1–2 mm) oval objects attached to the base of the hair.

    b. The lice themselves are difficult to find.

    c. Secondary changes in the scalp, including impetiginous changes and furuncles, often develop.

  2. Body (pediculosis corporis)

    a. The lice are rarely found on the skin, but may be present in clothing.

    b. Skin lesions are characterized by changes secondary to scratching and by secondary impetiginous lesions and furuncles.

  3. Genital or pubic region (phthiriasis inguinalis)

    a. The pubic hair characteristically is infested with nits.

    b. The lice are often difficult to find.

    c. Small black dots, which are probably excreta, may be seen.

IV. Laboratory studies None.

V. Differential diagnosis

  A. The presence of nits or mature lice is pathognomonic.

  B. The secondary lesions, including excoriations, impetigo, and furuncles, can be of multiple origins. Their location on the scalp, pubic areas, or the skin folds may be helpful in diagnosing pediculosis.

VI. Treatment Treatment involves the use of 1% gamma benzene hexachloride (Kwell), which is available as a shampoo, cream, and lotion:

  A. Pediculosis capitis (head lice) Shampoo with Kwell and leave on scalp for 5 minutes. Then rinse. Remove nits with fine tooth comb. Repeat once in 24 hours.

  B. Pediculosis corporis (body lice) Wash thoroughly with soap and water. Apply Kwell lotion or cream. Kill lice in clothing by boiling, dry cleaning, or using DDT (chlorophenothane), or a combination of these.

VII. Complications Secondary infection with impetigo, furuncles, or regional lymphadenitis, or a combination of these.

VIII. Consultation – referral Questions concerning diagnosis.

IX. Follow-up As needed.

PINWORMS (Pediatric and Adult)

I. **Definition**   Pinworms produce an infestation whose main symptom is anal itching. It is the most common parasitic infestation in children in the United States.

II. **Etiology**

   A. The intestinal nematode *Enterobius vermicularis.*

   B. Infestation begins with ingestion of eggs from fecally contaminated hands. Eggs mature during passage through the intestinal tract, and adults mate and females deposit thousands of eggs on the perineum after they migrate out from the anus. The life cycle is 15–28 days.

III. **Clinical features**

   A. **Symptoms**

   1. Patient may be asymptomatic, and the worms noticed fortuitous

   2. Primary symptom is anal pruritus.

   3. Pain may be present in the genital area of females.

   B. **Signs**

   1. Rectal examination may be normal.

   2. Perianal excoriation is present.

   3. Adult pinworms may be seen in the stool or on the perineum. Pinworms are approximately 1 cm in length and look like white thread.

IV. **Diagnostic studies**

   A. Observation of worms by a responsible person is sufficient for diagnosis.

   B. Examination for pinworm eggs will also establish the diagnosis:

   1. Press a piece of clear plastic tape directly over the anus and surrounding skin, preferably very early in the morning.

   2. Remove tape and place on glass slide with sticky side down.

   3. Lift tape and allow a drop of toluene to run between the tape and the slide.

   4. Examine microscopically under low power for the characteristic football-shaped eggs.

5. Examination of stool microscopically is not helpful since the eggs are deposited on the perianal skin.

C. Pinworms do not cause eosinophilia.

V. **Differential diagnosis**   Other causes of anal pruritus.

VI. **Treatment**

A. **General measures**

1. Stress personal hygiene, particularly hand washing before eating and after using the toilet.

2. Wash pajamas and bed linens of entire family in regular laundry detergent after treatment.

B. **Specific therapy**   Treat all family members at the same time:

1. Pyrantel pamoate (Antiminth) suspension given as a single oral dose of 1 ml per 5 kg (10 lb) of body weight. Maximum dose is 20 ml

   or

2. Mebendazole (Vermox), 1 chewable tablet for all weights, given as a single dose for children over 2 years of age and adults.

VII. **Complications**

A. Vulvovaginitis from migration to the vagina.

B. Secondary skin infection at sites of excoriation.

III. **Consultation – referral**   None in uncomplicated cases.

IX. **Follow-up**   Return visit only for recurrence.

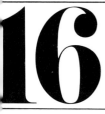 **Miscellaneous Infections**

MEASLES (Pediatric and Adult)

I. **Definition**   A highly contagious, febrile, exanthematous, viral disease associated with a high rate of serious complications.

II. **Etiology**   Measles virus.

III. **Clinical features**

A. **Symptoms**

1. The incubation period is 10–12 days.

2. The catarrhal, or prodromal, period before the rash lasts for 3–5 days:

a. The patient is usually very ill, with fever up to 104° F.

b. Coryza, cough, and conjunctivitis are prominent.

c. Marked malaise and anorexia are present.

d. Vomiting or diarrhea may occur.

3. The rash usually begins on the head and neck and spreads caudally, reaching the feet on the second or third day:

a. The fever and symptoms of the prodrome continue after the appearance of the rash, and symptoms are most severe as the rash reaches its peak.

b. By the second or third day of rash, the fever usually falls and symptoms begin to decrease.

c. Fever persisting after day 4 suggests the presence of complications.

B. **Signs**

1. Fever is present throughout the prodromal period, increasing in stepwise fashion until the height of the rash and rapidly declining on day 2 or 3 of the rash.

2. Marked nasal discharge, conjunctivitis, and pharyngeal infection begin prodromally and continue into the rash period.

3. Koplik's spots are pathognomonic and appear on the buccal mucosa two days before the appearance of the rash.

4. The maculopapular rash begins about the face and hairline and descends, gradually becoming confluent and eventually desquamating.

IV. Laboratory studies

A. Paired serum samples (from the acute and convalescent periods) should be drawn and sent to state laboratories for confirmation of diagnosis.

B. Other laboratory tests should be done on the basis of the presence of complications, after consultation.

V. Differential diagnosis

A. Rubella.

B. Roseola.

C. Rocky Mountain spotted fever.

D. Scarlet fever.

E. Enterovirus exanthems.

F. Drug rashes.

VI. Treatment

A. Prevention

1. Live measles vaccine should be given alone or as part of combined measles-mumps-rubella vaccine as soon as possible after a child is 1 year old.

2. Nonimmune persons exposed to measles should be given 0.25 ml per kilogram of body weight of gamma globulin not later than 5 days after exposure. Children over 1 year old should also be given live measles vaccine 8 weeks later.

B. Therapy

1. No specific therapy.

2. Isolation of patient from the onset of the catarrhal stage through the third day of the rash.

    3. Notification of appropriate public health authorities so control measures may be instituted. Be certain to confirm suspected cases.

    4. Investigation of immune status of family and immediate contacts, and appropriate steps to limit spread of measles with gamma globulin (see **VI.A.2**).

    5. Antipyretic therapy (see Chapter 5, Upper Respiratory Tract Infection [Common Cold] [Pediatric and Adult], **VI.C**).

    6. Antibiotic therapy only as indicated for specific complications.

    7. Adequate fluid and nutritional intake.

    8. Darkened room: This may be more comfortable, but is not necessary for conjunctivitis.

VII. Complications

A. Pneumonia

    1. Pneumonia may occur at anytime during the course of measles.

    2. It should be treated as bacterial pneumonia because it usually represents superimposed bacterial disease.

B. Otitis media

    1. This is a very common complication.

    2. It should be treated according to the guidelines in Chapter 5, Acute Purulent Otitis Media (Pediatric and Adult), **VI**.

C. Encephalitis

    1. This is a very serious complication occurring in 0.1% of cases.

    2. Onset is most commonly between two and six days after the onset of the rash.

D. Tuberculosis

    1. Tuberculin sensitivity is depressed during and immediately after measles.

    2. Inactive tuberculosis may be activated, and children with positive tuberculin tests should be on antituberculosis therapy.

VIII. Consultation – referral

A. Patients with evidence of encephalitis should be referred immediately.

B. Consultation is indicated for patients with pneumonia.

C. Patients who are known to have inactive tuberculosis should be referred.

D. Public health authorities should be notified when suspected cases are seen.

IX. **Follow-up**   All patients should be seen 3 or 4 days after the onset of the rash.

INFECTIOUS MONONUCLEOSIS (Pediatric and Adult)

I. **Definition**   A disease primarily of children and young adults character ized mainly by fever, sore throat, enlarged lymph nodes, malaise, and lassitude.

II. **Etiology**   Probably the Epstein-Barr virus (EBV).

III. **Clinical features**

A. Symptoms

1. Sore throat.

2. Malaise and lassitude.

3. Usually, *no* nasal congestion, earache, cough, or other symptoms commonly present in respiratory infections.

B. Signs

1. Fever (often $101^\circ - 103^\circ$ F).

2. Inflammation of the pharynx (often exudative).

3. Bilateral usually nontender enlargement of the lymph nodes. Th cervical lymph nodes are almost always involved; the axillary and inguinal nodes, frequently.

4. Often, splenomegaly.

5. Sometimes, erythematous maculopapular rash.

6. Periorbital edema.

7. Sometimes, jaundice.

IV. **Laboratory studies**

A. Throat culture is done to rule out streptococcal pharyngitis.

    B. White blood cell and differential count usually show lymphocytosis, with 10–20% atypical lymphocytes by the seventh day of illness.

    C. Heterophil antibody determination, or "MONO-Test," is usually positive.

V. Differential diagnosis

    A. Streptococcal pharyngitis.

    B. Hepatitis of other origin in patients in whom jaundice develops.

    C. Viral exanthems and other causes of skin rash.

    D. Other causes of cervical lymphadenopathy and splenomegaly that have negative heterophile, such as cytomegalovirus or toxoplasma infection.

VI. Treatment

    A. Take acetaminophen or aspirin for fever (see Chapter 5, Upper Respiratory Tract Infection [Common Cold] [Pediatric and Adult], **VI.C,** for dosage).

    B. Increase fluid intake.

    C. Rest according to degree of illness. Forced bedrest in mildly ill patient is *not* necessary.

    D. Do *not* give *ampicillin* for coexisting problems in patients with infectious mononucleosis, as a rash often develops.

VII. Complications

    A. Hepatitis.

    B. Ruptured spleen.

    C. Hemolytic anemia.

    D. Aseptic meningitis.

    E. Polyneuritis.

VIII. Consultation – referral

    A. Splenomegaly.

    B. Tender spleen.

    C. Jaundice.

    D. Marked tonsillar enlargement with difficulty in swallowing.

    E. Nervous system involvement.

    F. Illness persisting for more than 2 weeks.

IX. **Follow-up**   Weekly until patient has recovered.

MUMPS (Pediatric and Adult)

I. **Definition**   Mumps is a clinical syndrome characterized by acute salivary gland enlargement, particularly of the parotid gland.

II. **Etiology**

    A. Mumps is usually caused by mumps virus, a member of the myxovirus family.

    B. Other myxoviruses, particularly the parainfluenza viruses, can cause clinical mumps and may account for second cases of mumps and for mumps in immunized children.

III. **Clinical features**

    A. **Symptoms**

       1. Incubation period lasts from 14–21 days, with an average of 18 days.

       2. Fever may precede development of parotid swelling by 1 or 2 days.

       3. Constitutional symptoms include headache, lethargy, anorexia, myalgia, and vomiting.

       4. Parotitis produces pain anterior to the ear, which is increased by eating, local pressure, and jaw movement and is accompanied by visible swelling.

       5. Symptoms related to complications (see **VII**) may *precede,* accompany, or follow parotitis.

    B. **Signs**

       1. Fever is present.

       2. Upper respiratory symptoms may accompany illness.

       3. Parotid swelling is characteristic:

          a. The swelling is diffuse and difficult to demarcate.

          b. Twenty-five percent of cases have unilateral involvement.

    c. The swelling obliterates the angle of the mandible and is usually maximal near the earlobe.

    d. Stensen's duct may be inflamed.

    e. There is marked variation in the amount of parotid swelling seen with mumps.

    f. Other salivary glands may be involved.

  4. Complications, particularly meningoencephalitis and orchitis (see **VII.A** and **C**), are common and should be looked for.

IV. Laboratory studies   None.

V. Differential diagnosis

A. Parotitis may be confused with the following:

  1. Anterior, cervical, or preauricular lymphadenitis.

  2. Idiopathic recurrent parotitis.

  3. Parotid duct stone with secondary infection.

  4. Mikulicz's syndrome — painless bilateral enlargement of the salivary and lacrimal glands, usually with dryness of the mouth and absence of tears.

B. Meningoencephalitis may occur with or without parotid swelling and must be distinguished from other causes of meningitis.

VI. Treatment

A. Prevention

  1. A live mumps virus vaccine may be given alone or as combined measles-mumps-rubella vaccine after 1 year of age. This is particularly recommended for persons approaching puberty and adult males with no history of mumps.

  2. Exposed postpuberal males with no history of natural mumps or immunization should be given live mumps vaccine.

  3. The value of gamma globulin is not established and it is not recommended.

B. Therapy

  1. No specific treatment.

  2. Analgesic and antipyretics: Acetaminophen or aspirin (see Chap-

ter 5, Upper Respiratory Tract Infection [Common Cold] [Pediatric and Adult], **VI.C**, for dosage).

3. Supportive care as required for specific complications.

4. Isolation: Mumps is contagious from as much as 7 days before to 9 days after parotid swelling is evident.

VII. Complications

A. Meningoencephalitis

1. This is a very common and usually benign complication.

2. It usually follows parotitis by 3–10 days, but may precede or occur in absence of parotitis.

3. Hospitalization for symptomatic care may be necessary in severe cases.

B. Nerve deafness is usually unilateral, occurring after mumps.

C. Orchitis

1. Orchitis is usually unilateral, occurring in postpuberal males.

2. There is marked variation in the severity of symptoms. Gonadal enlargement and pain, fever, headache, nausea and vomiting, and abdominal pain all may occur.

3. Impotence does not result and sterility is extremely rare.

D. Pancreatitis is uncommon but can be severe.

VIII. Consultation – referral   All patients with evidence of complications should be discussed with physician.

IX. Follow-up

A. Patients with complications should be checked in 24 hours, at least by telephone. Continue close follow-up until there is improvement.

B. Follow-up is not required in uncomplicated cases.

ROSEOLA INFANTUM (EXANTHEMA SUBITUM) (Pediatric)

I. **Definition**   Roseola infantum is an acute, benign febrile illness limited exclusively to children from 6 months to 3 years of age and characteriz cessation of fever as a rash appears.

II. **Etiology**   Unknown, but presumably a virus.

III. Clinical features

A. Symptoms

1. High fever of sudden onset lasts from 1—5 days, usually 3 or 4 days. Fever may be sustained or intermittent.

2. There is a marked contrast between the high fever and the paucity of symptoms.

3. Symptoms, usually minimal, may include malaise, vomiting, and coryza.

4. Fever and the other minimal symptoms clear with the onset of the rash.

5. The degree of contagiousness and the incubation period are not known.

B. Signs

1. Fever occurs prior to the onset of the rash.

2. Minimal coryza, slight injection of the pharynx, and cervical and occipital adenopathy are the only clinical findings prior to the rash.

3. Rash occurs with lysis of fever:

   a. Faint maculopapular rash first occurs on the trunk and neck, with minimal involvement of the upper face and the extremities.

   b. The rash usually clears in 24—48 hours.

IV. Laboratory studies   If a rash is not present and fever is the only abnormal finding, perform urinalysis and urine culture to rule out urinary tract infection.

V. Differential diagnosis

A. Urinary tract infection before onset of rash.

B. Rubella.

C. Other acute febrile illnesses.

VI. Treatment

A. Prevention: None.

B. Therapy

     1. No specific treatment.

     2. Antipyretic therapy with acetaminophen or aspirin (see Chapter Upper Respiratory Tract Infection [Common Cold] [Pediatric and Adult], **VI.C.1**, for dosage).

VII. **Complications**   Febrile seizures.

VIII. **Consultation – referral**

  A. Seizures.

  B. Fever

     1. Lasting more than 4 days.

     2. Continuing after rash develops.

     3. Associated with more than the minimal symptoms (see **III.A**).

IX. **Follow-up**   Maintain daily contact with family until diagnosis is confirmed.

RUBELLA (Pediatric and Adult)

I. **Definition**   Postnatally acquired rubella is a usually mild disease associated with a 3-day rash and lymph node enlargement. Congenital infections are associated with a high incidence of congenital malformations.

II. **Etiology**   Rubella virus.

III. **Clinical features**

  A. **Symptoms**

     1. Incubation period lasts 14–21 days.

     2. Transmission is by droplet spread or direct contact with infected persons or by exposure to material freshly contaminated by nasopharyngeal secretions, feces, or urine.

     3. Prodromal symptoms either are absent or consist of minimal lethargy, anorexia, and upper respiratory tract symptoms.

  B. **Signs**

     1. The maculopapular rash begins about the face and neck, with rapid spread to the trunk and extremities. It usually disappears by the third day, with slight desquamation occasionally occurring

     2. Generalized lymphadenopathy is usually most pronounced in the suboccipital, postauricular, and cervical nodes.

3. Fever is usually of low grade or absent during the period of the rash.

IV. Laboratory studies

A. Paired serum samples separated by a 2-week interval should be submitted to the state laboratory for confirmation of the diagnosis if the patient has been in contact with pregnant women. A fourfold rise in the **hemagglutination inhibition titer** confirms the diagnosis.

B. Pregnant women whose immunity to rubella is unknown and who have contact with a suspected case of rubella should have a **rubella titer drawn** *immediately*. A titer of greater than 1:10 indicates immunity and the individual can be reassured that she is immune. A second blood specimen 4 weeks later should be obtained in individuals with titers of 1:10 or less. A fourfold rise in titer in a previously nonimmune individual documents infection, and the pregnant woman should be referred to a physician for a decision regarding possible termination of pregnancy.

V. Differential diagnosis

A. Measles.

B. Scarlet fever.

C. Roseola.

D. Infectious mononucleosis.

E. Enteroviral exanthems.

F. Drug rashes.

VI. Treatment

A. Prevention

1. Rubella vaccine should be given at 1 year of age either combined with measles or as combined measles-mumps-rubella vaccine.

2. Emphasis should be placed on ensuring that all females in the child-bearing age or approaching puberty are immune. A single hemagglutination inhibition titer of greater than 1:10 establishes immunity. Nonimmune females should receive rubella vaccine and must use a medically acceptable method for pregnancy prevention for 2 months following immunization.

3. The use of serum immune globulin is *not* recommended, but may be considered for those who will not consider therapeutic abortion.

B. Treatment

1. No specific treatment is available.

2. Antipyretic therapy may be used, but is rarely necessary (see Chapter 5, Upper Respiratory Tract Infection [Common Cold] [Pediatric and Adult], **VI.C**, for dosage).

3. Contacts should be evaluated to determine if pregnant women are at risk.

4. Patient should be isolated while rash is present.

5. Cases should be reported to the appropriate public health authorities.

VII. Complications

A. Severe damage to the fetus if the infection occurs in a pregnant individual.

B. Polyarthralgia and polyarthritis can occur in adults following both natural disease and immunization.

C. Encephalitis is rare.

VIII. Consultation — referral

A. Consultation for all patients with complications.

B. Consultation for exposure of nonimmune pregnant women.

IX. Follow-up

A. Follow-up is not needed in uncomplicated cases in which there is no exposure of nonimmune pregnant women.

B. Follow-up is needed to obtain convalescent serum samples from patient and exposed nonimmune pregnant women to confirm the diagnosis of rubella so that appropriate steps may be taken to terminate pregnancy, if desired.

VARICELLA (CHICKENPOX) (Pediatric and Adult)

I. **Definition**   An acute, usually benign, highly contagious disease of childhood associated with a pruritic vesicular rash.

II. **Etiology**   Varicella-zoster virus causes both chickenpox and herpes zoster.

III. Clinical features

A. Symptoms

1. The incubation period ranges from 10—21 days, with an average of 14—16 days.

2. A prodrome is usually absent in children; adolescents may have 1 or 2 days of prodromal fever, malaise, and anorexia.

3. Rash is characterized as follows:

   a. Lesions appear in crops, with rapid evolution (in 6—8 hours) of individual lesions from macule to papule to vesicle to crusting. Lesions in all stages are present at the same time in any given area.

   b. Lesions begin on the trunk and spread peripherally, with least involvement of the extremities.

   c. Oral mucous membranes frequently are involved with vesicles that ulcerate.

   d. Rash is usually very pruritic.

   e. New lesions usually occur for 3—5 days.

4. Onset of fever is usually at the time of the rash, and its severity is proportional to the degree of skin involvement of the rash.

5. Headache, malaise, and anorexia are usually related to the height of the fever.

B. Signs   Major physical findings are related to the rash (see **III.A.3**).

IV. Laboratory studies   None.

V. Differential diagnosis

A. Diagnosis usually is not a problem.

B. Chickenpox may be confused with the following:

1. Herpesvirus hominis infections.

2. Generalized vaccinia (history of exposure important).

3. Smallpox (history of exposure important).

4. Drug eruptions.

5. Impetigo.

6. Secondary syphilis.

7. Erythema multiforme.

8. Hand-foot-and-mouth disease (Coxsackie virus).

VI. Treatment

A. Prevention

1. No vaccine is available.

2. Regular gamma globulin is not effective in preventing disease.

3. If exposed to varicella, patients receiving steroid or immunosup-pressive therapy, patients with immunologic disorders or malignant disease, and newborns should be referred for consideration for zoster immune globulin (ZIG).

B. Therapy

1. Symptomatic care for skin

   a. Fingernails should be kept short to minimize excoriation and scarring by scratching.

   b. Drying lotion (calamine) may be applied to lesions to decrea: pruritus.

   c. Soap and water washing does not spread virus and does reduc secondary infection.

2. **Antipyretic**   Tylenol or aspirin (see Chapter 5, Upper Respirato Tract Infection [Common Cold] [Pediatric and Adult], **VI.C**, for dosage).

3. **Isolation**   The disease is contagious until the lesions have cruste

VII. Complications

A. **Secondary bacterial infections** (streptococcal or staphylococcal, or both).

B. **Pneumonia**   Primary viral pneumonia is extremely rare as a compli cation in children but relatively common in adults.

C. **Encephalitis** is a rare complication that has a better prognosis than most postinfectious encephalitides.

D. **Severe disseminated disease** may occur in newborns, patients receiv steroid or immunosuppressive therapy, or patients with immunologic deficiency or malignant disease.

E. **Bleeding disorders** occur very rarely.

VIII. **Consultation – referral**

A. All patients with conditions predisposing to severe disseminated disease (see **VII.D**), immediately upon exposure to chickenpox for consideration for zoster immune globulin.

B. Development of pneumonia, bleeding problems, or central nervous system symptoms.

C. Severe secondary bacterial infections.

IX. **Follow-up**

A. In routine cases no follow-up is required.

B. Patient should return in 48 hours if there is concern about secondary bacterial infection.

Index

Note To avoid unnecessary repetition of the major outline headings in the text (i.e., definition, etiology, clinical features, laboratory studies, differential diagnosis, treatment, complications, consultation-referral, and follow-up), these headings have not all been indexed under specific diseases and disorders. Rather, only inclusive page numbers for a disease or disorder are given, followed by subentries for lengthy, major discussions on these pages.